Demystifying Interventional Radiology

Sriharsha Athreya • Mahmood Albahhar

Editors

Demystifying Interventional Radiology

A Guide for Medical Students

Second Edition

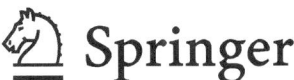 Springer

Editors
Sriharsha Athreya
Interventional Radiology
McMaster University
Hamilton, ON, Canada

Mahmood Albahhar
Interventional Radiology
McMaster University
Hamilton, ON, Canada

ISBN 978-3-031-12022-0   ISBN 978-3-031-12023-7   (eBook)
https://doi.org/10.1007/978-3-031-12023-7

This Springer imprint is published by the registered company Springer Nature Switzerland AG
The registered company address is: Gewerbestrasse 11, 6330 Cham, Switzerland

Acknowledgments

I am extremely grateful to everyone who have contributed in bringing this book to print. My sincere thanks to the many medical students who supported the concept of this book on interventional radiology and to all the authors whose contributions helped pull this book together. I wish to thank our partners in industry for allowing us to use images of the equipment in the book. Your assistance is truly appreciated.

Finally, special gratitude to my parents, my wife, and two sons for being so patient, understanding, and supportive of me in this and all my endeavors.

Contents

Part III   Common Interventional Radiology Procedures

Part I
Introduction

Chapter 1
Interventional Radiology: The Early Days and Innovation

Jason Martin and Ashis Bagchee-Clark

The Beginning

For some, the birthplace of interventional radiology (IR) can be considered the Karolinska Institute in Sweden. There, in 1953, Swedish radiologist Dr. Sven Ivar Seldinger introduced the technique of using a hollow needle to puncture and gain access to a blood vessel, inserting an exchange wire through the hollow of this needle into the vessel, and then using this exchange wire to introduce medical devices such as catheters [1]. The eponymously named Seldinger technique was what allowed many early angiographers to expand their field of practice. Today, the Seldinger technique remains a commonly used technique across interventional radiology.

Ten years later, in 1963, American vascular radiologist Dr. Charles Dotter was conducting an abdominal aortogram in an individual who presented with renal artery stenosis when Dotter realized he had recanalized a right artery occlusion by simply passing the catheter through the occlusion [2]. Dotter reported his findings at the Czechoslovak Radiological Congress in June that year, where he spoke openly about the potential therapeutic promise of the catheter [2]. Seven months later, Dotter performed the first known intentional transluminal percutaneous angioplasty on a woman named Laura Shaw [2]. For many others, this case can be considered the birth of interventional radiology, and Charles Dotter is considered by many the "father" of interventional radiology.

J. Martin
Department of Medical Imaging, University of Toronto, Toronto, ON, Canada
e-mail: jason.martin@medportal.ca

A. Bagchee-Clark (✉)
Michael G. DeGroote School of Medicine, McMaster University, Hamilton, ON, Canada
e-mail: ashis.bagcheeclark@medportal.ca

During his presentation in Czechoslovakia, Dotter discussed catheter biopsy, controlled catheterization, occlusion catheterization, and the basis for catheter end-arterectomy [3]. He urged a change in paradigm, envisioning the diagnostic catheter as a means for delivering novel therapy. This radical shift was a shock for many, as angiographers at the time were trained to help referring clinical colleagues with diagnosis, not treat patients themselves with percutaneous methods.

Dotter led the charge: a paper published by Dotter and Melvin Judkins (his trainee at the time) in the November 1964 issue of *Circulation* outlined their 5-month experience with angioplasty [4]. It detailed the treatment of 11 extremities in 9 patients, including 4 short SFA occlusions and 4 long SFA occlusions. While not all the procedures were successful, four out of seven scheduled amputations were averted. Dotter's experience continued to grow, and in 1966 he reported treatment outcomes of 82 lesions in 74 patients, including 6 iliac artery stenoses. This experience allowed Dotter to refine his technique, decreasing the size of dilation catheters and improving their design. Two years later, he reported 217 dilations of 153 lesions in 127 patients [5], with excellent results.

The term "interventional radiology" was coined by Alexander Margulis (a gastrointestinal radiologist) in an editorial in the *American Journal of Roentgenology* in 1967. At the time, radiologists worldwide were exploring the treatment of non-vascular disease through percutaneous methods. This included treatment of frozen shoulders by joint distension during arthrography, abscess drainage, intrauterine transfusion of the fetus under fluoroscopic guidance, pulmonary and liver biopsies, and transjugular cholangiography. Margulis realized that a new specialty was developing and, in his editorial, defined IR and also set requirements for its performance. Central to IR training was the need for specific training, technical skills, clinical education, and the ability to care for patients before, during, and after the procedure.

Dotter was not enthralled with the term "interventional," as he thought it would generate confusion among the public and physicians about what IR could do. However, the term allowed for the creation of a new field and the semantic and conceptual separation from general diagnostic radiology and its subspecialties.

1960s–1980s

The mid-1960s–1980s were a time of great development for radiology, as Dotter's work challenged the knowledge of diagnostic angiographers and spurred their transition to interventionalists. In the earlier years, new techniques were often introduced to clinical practice without experimental and patient safety testing. Many emergencies in clinical medicine forced radiologists to innovate, creating new procedures and techniques to combat a variety of pathology. Arterial embolization of upper gastrointestinal bleeding was a major advancement created in this manner. The application of experience and techniques in one organ system to a different system led to new indications for interventional procedures. As newer techniques were developed, detailed experimental testing in animals was performed before introduction to clinical use, promoting the use of ethical innovation and patient care, as well as evidence-based medicine.

Percutaneous Transluminal Angioplasty

After his successful first procedures, Dotter began to recruit patients for percutaneous transluminal angioplasty (PTA) mainly from general practitioners and internists. Surgeons were not interested in nonsurgical treatment of atherosclerotic disease and were adamantly opposed to PTA. Through media advertising, Dotter was able to attract patients interested in angioplasty. Admitted to the hospital under radiology, residents and fellows worked them up and prepared them for PTA. An article in *Life* earned Dotter the nickname of "Crazy Charlie," and this media attention garnered a VIP patient, the wife of the owner of a large international company in New York City. Dotter flew to New York with his team and performed PTA of the patient's SFA stenosis successfully. The patient and her family donated $500,000 to the Oregon Health and Science University radiology department, which allowed Dotter to purchase angiographic equipment and perform PTA more efficiently.

Although Dotter published extensively on PTA in the first 4 years, PTA procedures in the United States were performed mostly in Portland. Angiographers in other institutions did not share Dotter's idea of intervention, choosing to focus on diagnosis. European angiographers were more progressive at that time, wanting to expand their scope of practice. Werner Porstmann, a friend of Dotter's from Berlin, started performing PTA in the 1960s, and Van Andel from the Netherlands modified the dilation catheters. The most credit goes to Eberhart Zeitler from Germany. His work resulted in European angiographers embracing PTA and treating patients with percutaneous techniques [6, 7]. In fact, German radiologist Andreas Gruentzig became interested in IR after hearing a speech by Zeitler on Dotter's method [8]. Andreas Gruentzig created a polyvinyl chloride balloon catheter in 1974, which revolutionized PTA [9]. Realizing the potential in these catheters, medical device manufacturers promoted balloon catheters avidly, and balloon PTA became popular. Gruentzig performed the first successful balloon dilations of coronary arteries in 1976 [10].

The success of PTA in Europe sparked the interest and creativity of angiographers in North America. Visiting Europe to see Gruentzig at work, some even stayed for fellowships. When they returned, they brought back these improved PTA procedures to the United States, where it began 15 years prior. With the rapid utilization of PTA in the United States, it became the most performed IR procedure in the country.

The Modern Age

In the decades following Seldinger and Dotter initiating the emergence of a new medical specialty, IR has evolved into a prominent department in practically every major modern hospital. To that point, 10% of all radiologists in the United States can be considered interventionalists [11]. The expansion of the specialty has brought with it a more exhaustive range of different diseases and conditions for which IR can be used. As an example, IR, originally a radiology subspecialty, has grown to the point where it has its own subspecialties, such as interventional oncology. Table 1.1 outlines numerous advancements made over the years in the field of IR [12–14]. Throughout this guide, an exploration of the modern landscape of IR will be undertaken.

Table 1.1 Milestones pioneered by interventional radiologists

1964	Angioplasty
1966	Embolization therapy to treat tumors and spinal cord vascular malformations
1967	Judkins technique of coronary angiography
1967	Closure of patent ductus arteriosus
1967	Selective vasoconstriction infusions for hemorrhage
1969	Catheter-delivered stenting technique and prototype stent
1960–1974	Tools for intervention such as heparinized guide wires and contrast injectors
1970s	Percutaneous removal of common bile duct stones
1970s	Occlusive coils
1972	Selective arterial embolization for GI bleeding
1973	Embolization for pelvic trauma
1974	Selective arterial thrombolysis for arterial occlusions
1974	Transhepatic embolization for variceal bleeding
1977–1978	Embolization technique for pulmonary arteriovenous malformations and varicoceles
1977–1983	Chemoembolization for treatment of hepatocellular carcinoma and disseminated liver metastases
1980	Cryoablation for liver tumors
1980s	Biliary stents to divert liver flow
1981	Embolization for splenic trauma
1982	TIPS (transjugular intrahepatic portosystemic shunt)
1982	Dilators for interventional urology and percutaneous removal of renal stones
1983	Balloon-expandable stent
1985	Self-expanding stents
1990s	Embolization of bone and kidney tumors, uterine artery embolization
1990s	RFA for soft tissue tumors
1991	Abdominal aortic stent grafts
1994	Balloon-expandable coronary stent
1995	Uterine artery embolization

Table 1.1 (continued)

1964	Angioplasty
1997	Intra-arterial delivery of tumor-killing viruses and gene therapy vectors to the liver
1999	Percutaneous transplantation of islet cells to the liver for diabetes
1999	Endovenous laser ablation to treat varicose veins
2000	Microwave ablation for renal tumors
2000	Prostatic artery embolization for benign prostatic hyperplasia

References

1. Higgs ZC, Macafee DA, Braithwaite BD, Maxwell-Armstrong CA. The Seldinger technique: 50 years on. Lancet. 2005;366(9494):1407–9.
2. Payne MM. Charles Theodore Dotter: the father of intervention. Tex Heart Inst J. 2001;28(1):28.
3. Dotter CT. Cardiac catheterization and angiographic techniques of the future. Cesk Radiol. 1965;19:217–36.
4. Dotter CT, Judkins MP. Transluminal treatment of atherosclerotic obstructions: description of a new technique and preliminary report of its applications. Circulation. 1964;30:654–70.
5. Dotter CT, Judkins MP, Rösch J. Nichtoperative, transluminale behandlung der arteriosklerotischenverschlussaffektionen. Fortschr Rontgenstr. 1968;109:125–33.
6. Zeitler E, Müller R. Erste egebnisse mit der katheter-rekanalisation nach dotter bei arteriellerverschlusskran- kenheit. Fortschr Rontgenstr. 1969;111:345–52.
7. Zeitler E, Schoop W, Schmidtkte I. Mechanische bchandlung von becken- arterienstenosen mitder perkutanen kathetertechnik. Verh Dtsch Kreislaufforsch. 1971;37:402–7.
8. Barton M, Grüntzig J, Husmann M, Rösch J. Balloon angioplasty–the legacy of Andreas Grüntzig, MD (1939–1985). Front Cardiovasc Med. 2014;1:15.
9. Grüntzig A, Hopff H. Percutane Recanalization chronischer arterieller verschlüsse mit einemneuen dilatation-skatheter. Dtsch Med Wochenschr. 1974;99:2502–5.
10. Grüntzig A. Percutane dilatation von koronarstenoses. Beschreibung eines neuen kathetersystem. Klin Wochenschr. 1976;54:543–5.
11. Sunshine JH, Lewis RS, Bhargavan M. A portrait of interventional radiologists in the United States. Am J Roentgenol. 2005;185(5):1103–12.
12. Rösch J, Keller FS, Kaufman JA. The birth, early years, and future of interventional radiology. J Vasc Interv Radiol. 2003;14(7):841–53.
13. Carnevale FC, Antunes AA, da Motta Leal Filho JM, de Oliveira Cerri LM, Baroni RH, Marcelino AS, Freire GC, Moreira AM, Srougi M, Cerri GG. Prostatic artery embolization as a primary treatment for benign prostatic hyperplasia: preliminary results in two patients. Cardiovasc Intervent Radiol. 2010;33(2):355–61.
14. Gupta JK, Sinha A, Lumsden MA, Hickey M. Uterine artery embolization for symptomatic uterine fibroids. Cochrane Database Syst Rev. 2014;12

Chapter 2
Basic X-Ray Physics

Anna Hwang, Prasaanthan Gopee-Ramanan, and Sandra Reis

X-Ray Production

Interventional radiology procedures allow an interventional radiologist with highly specialized training to utilize the imaging function of a fluoroscopy system to carry out diagnostic and therapeutic procedures for a wide variety of diseases and conditions. X-ray production with a fluoroscopy unit happens much in the same way as a conventional radiography unit. Within an X-ray tube, by colliding electrons produced at high velocity from a cathode (negatively charged metal) with the atoms of the anode (a positively charged metal such as tungsten-rhenium alloy and molybdenum), energy is released in the form of X-ray photons. A key property of X-rays that differentiates them from other types of radiation is the fact that since X-rays are not particles and do not have an electrical charge, they have greater penetration power, making them effective for imaging the body [1, 2]. The voltage supplied to the cathode and the numbers of electrons emitted toward the anode over a time period are the kilovolt peak (kVp) and milliampere-seconds (mAs), respectively.

A. Hwang (✉)
Michael G. DeGroote School of Medicine, McMaster University, Hamilton, ON, Canada
e-mail: anna.hwang@medportal.ca

P. Gopee-Ramanan
Department of Radiology, Michael G. DeGroote School of Medicine, Faculty of Health Sciences, McMaster University, Hamilton, ON, Canada
e-mail: prasa.gopee@medportal.ca

S. Reis
Diagnostic Imaging, St. Joseph's Healthcare Hamilton, Hamilton, ON, Canada
e-mail: sreis@stjosham.on.ca

© The Author(s), under exclusive license to Springer Nature Switzerland AG 2022
S. Athreya, M. Albahhar (eds.), *Demystifying Interventional Radiology*, https://doi.org/10.1007/978-3-031-12023-7_2

X-Ray Interactions with Biological Tissues

The intensity of an X-ray beam decreases as it interacts with matter, due to absorption or scattering. As the X-ray photons pass through tissue, they encounter atomic electrons. Upon interaction with an electron, a photon's energy can be absorbed by the electron (photoelectric absorption), or the photon can be scattered in a different direction (Compton scattering) [1, 2].

Photoelectric absorption is key to generating the image. Different materials have different propensities for beam absorption, producing image contrast. In general, beam absorption increases with the thickness, density, and atomic number of a material. For example, since bone is more dense and has a higher atomic number than soft tissue, bone absorbs more of the X-ray beam and appears brighter than soft tissue on the radiographic image. Air absorbs very little of the X-ray beam, so it appears darker in the image.

Compton scattering, on the other hand, dampens image quality, but is an unavoidable by-product of X-ray imaging.

However, both photoelectric absorption and Compton scattering generate damaging ions in tissue. If an electron absorbs enough energy from a photon, it can be ejected from an atom. Ejected electrons can damage DNA directly or react with other molecules, such as water, to generate free radicals. Free radicals are highly reactive and cause damage to DNA and other cell constituents [3, 4]. The biological effects of ionizing radiation can be classified as either somatic or genetic.

Somatic Effects

Somatic effects manifest in the irradiated individual. Stochastic effects (e.g., cancers) occur in keeping with the linear no-threshold (LNT) model, where there is no threshold dose for damage to occur, but higher doses increase the probability of disease. Deterministic effects (e.g., cataracts) occur depending on how much cumulative radiation dose a person has received [4]. Examples include:

- Cancer—leukemia, thyroid, breast, lung, gastrointestinal, skin
- Skin effects—erythema, desquamation, hair loss
- Gastrointestinal epithelia—sloughing off negatively impacting digestion and nutrient absorption
- Bone marrow—anemia, immunosuppression
- Lung tissue—radiation pneumonitis, pulmonary fibrosis, mesothelioma

Genetic Effects

Genetic and teratogenic effects do not yield observable effects in the irradiated individual, but rather in his or her offspring. Genetic effects are those passed on from parent to child as a result of point mutations, single-stranded breaks, or double-stranded breaks in germline cells impacting the future development of the progeny [4]. Teratogenic effects occur when a developing fetus is exposed to radiation and manifest as:

- Childhood cancer
- Microcephaly
- Poorly formed eyes
- Slow growth
- Mental retardation

Acknowledgments We would like to thank Prasaanthan Gopee-Ramanan and Sandra Reis for their contributions to this chapter (information given on first page of chapter).

References

1. Carlton RR, Adler AM, Balac V. Principles of radiographic imaging: an art and a science. 6th ed. Cengage Learning, Inc.; 2018.
2. Dixon R, Whitlow C. The physical basis of diagnostic imaging. In: Chen M, Pope T, Ott D, editors. Basic radiology. 2nd ed. North Carolina: McGraw-Hill; 2010.
3. Government of Canada, H. C. H. E. A. C. P. S. B. Safety code 35: radiation protection in radiology—Large facilities; 2008. p. 1–88.
4. Kelsey CA, Heintz PH, Sandoval DJ, Chambers GD, Adolphi NL, Paffett KS. Radiation biology of medical imaging. Wiley, Incorporated; 2014.

Chapter 3
Principles of Radiation Safety in Interventional Radiology

Anna Hwang, Prasaanthan Gopee-Ramanan, and Sandra Reis

X-Ray Equipment in Interventional Radiology

In a fluoroscopy system, typically a C-arm in interventional radiology, X-ray photons emitted by the X-ray tube pass through the table and the patient's body and then are received by the flat panel detector. The flat panel detector converts the X-ray signal into binary electrical energy by means of analog-to-digital converters (ADCs). Commercial or vendor-specific software then makes use of the raw data to display an image on the computer monitor (Fig. 3.1) [1, 2].

Radiation Safety in Interventional Radiology

To understand the principles of radiation safety, one must consider the concept of radiation dose or exposure in greater detail. Since X-rays are ionizing radiation, there is the potential for damage to body tissues resulting from excessive exposure.

A. Hwang (✉)
Michael G. DeGroote School of Medicine, McMaster University, Hamilton, ON, Canada
e-mail: anna.hwang@medportal.ca

P. Gopee-Ramanan
Department of Radiology, Michael G. DeGroote School of Medicine, Faculty of Health Sciences, McMaster University, Hamilton, ON, Canada
e-mail: prasa.gopee@medportal.ca

S. Reis
Diagnostic Imaging, St. Joseph's Healthcare Hamilton, Hamilton, ON, Canada
e-mail: sreis@stjosham.on.ca

S. Athreya, M. Albahhar (eds.), *Demystifying Interventional Radiology*,
https://doi.org/10.1007/978-3-031-12023-7_3

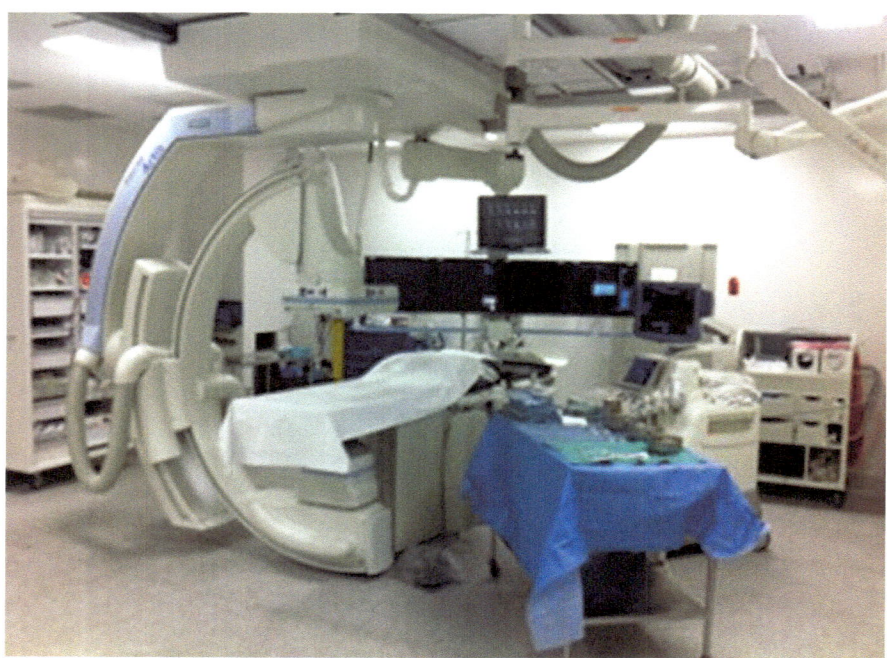

Fig. 3.1 Modern IR suite depicting fluoroscopy C-arm, ultrasound equipment, and sterile tray setup [original image]

Thus, one of the key aims of radiologists, technologists, physicists, engineers, and regulators is to keep radiation exposure or dose to all personnel and patients as low as reasonably achievable—referred to as the ALARA principle [3].

There has been great emphasis in the last few years regarding ionizing radiation and the cumulative doses received by patients who are subjected to a high volume of diagnostic examinations, procedures, and treatments for various disease processes. All modern X-ray equipment can produce detailed dose reports in milligrays (mGy) that in turn become a permanent part of the patient's record. This tool has proved to be invaluable to monitor high-risk patients and to contribute to quality assurance programs established within the individual department. Some patients keep a personal record of X-ray exposure/dose for their own purposes. It is our professional and personal goal to minimize radiation exposure to the patient without affecting the quality of the diagnostic procedure.

Reducing radiation dose to patients will result in a proportional decrease in the scatter dose received by the staff in radiology. Minimizing patient and occupational dose involves three cardinal variables: time, distance, and shielding.

Time

To decrease the amount of time X-rays are being produced, the following steps can be taken [1, 3]:

- Pulsed mode should be used whenever possible to reduce the number of fractions of a second a beam is being produced.
- Fluoroscopy should only be used to observe objects or structures that are in motion. Review of the LIH (last-image hold) should be used for study, consultation, and educational purposes, eliminating the need for extended radiation exposure.
- The exposure times should be limited according to the patient's age and gender as well as the potential for subsequent examinations and further exposure.
- For DSA (digital subtraction angiography), frame rates can be set according to the body part being imaged. Areas that exhibit fast flow rates such as the aorta will have higher frame rates in comparison to slower flow rates in the extremities.
- The use of X-ray delays can significantly reduce radiation exposure. The X-ray will not expose until a determined amount of time has lapsed to eliminate nondiagnostic images. As a team, the technologist, radiologist, and associated staff should review fluoroscopy time and dose values on a regular basis to chart trends and evaluate departmental performance.
- Supportive imaging modalities or options, like ultrasound, last-image hold (LIH), and tailored frame rates in DSA, should be utilized whenever possible to avoid the need for continuous fluoroscopic image acquisition.
- Pre-procedure imaging to define the relevant anatomy and pathology should be used to plan the procedure. These images can be imported and displayed in the examination room for a fast and effective reference.

Distance

The intensity of the X-ray beam decreases in a manner proportional to the distance squared from the source. As a rule, if you double the distance, you reduce the exposure by a factor of four. If the distance is tripled, exposure is reduced by a factor of nine [1, 3].

- Have all nonessential personnel stand at least 3 m from the X-ray collimator on the C-arm.
- For the patient's safety, the closer the flat panel detector is brought to the body part being imaged, the farther the X-ray source will be.
- Hands should be kept outside of the radiation field: extension tubing should be used for injections, and power injectors should be utilized when possible to eliminate or reduce the exposure.
- During power injections, the staff should vacate the examination room and observe the patient through the lead-lined windows.

Shielding

Shielding can be thought of as the final barrier available to block unnecessary or scatter radiation within the examination room [1, 3].

- It is imperative that a full lead apron and thyroid collar are worn during all fluoroscopic examinations. Lead is an excellent attenuator of X-rays due to its high density and high atomic number. Lead aprons contain 0.5 mm of lead and are an optimal combination of lightness and protection. Alternatively, metals such as tin and tungsten can be used, as these also have excellent attenuation abilities. Polyvinyl chloride is used in new-generation aprons to give the apron increased flexibility and durability.
- Ceiling-suspended shields and lead under the table drapes can provide additional dose reduction especially to the head and neck and lower extremities.
- If hands must be placed underneath the beam, lead gloves must be worn.
- Lead-lined eyewear is recommended if shields are not readily available.
- Irradiation of the patient's gonads (ovaries and testes) should be avoided if possible; otherwise the gonads must be shielded to prevent germline mutations.

Further Recommendations

Apart from the cardinal triad of time, distance, and shielding, several resources offer up further means of reducing radiation dose [1, 3]:

Technical Considerations:
- The edges of the X-ray beam should be observed on all images to make sure that only the target areas were irradiated.
- The X-ray beam must be well collimated to reduce radiation that does not contribute to the image.
- Grids should be placed between the patient and the image detector to filter scattered photons.
- Use the highest X-ray tube voltage possible without compromising image quality, as this reduces the amount of absorption and scatter in the tissue.
- Monitor, and increase whenever possible, X-ray tube filtration to eliminate low-energy X-ray photons, which contribute to radiation dose but not to the quality of the image.
- Reduce the use of magnification mode as much as possible since it increases tube current, thereby producing more X-ray photons capable of contributing to dose.
- Reposition tube for long procedures to avoid irradiating a single area for a prolonged period of time. This will reduce the incidence and impact of radiation injury to the skin, which can cause erythema, itching, and peeling as well as increase the risk for skin cancers.

Additional Safety Recommendations:

- Be especially vigilant to reduce X-ray exposure of the eyes and thyroid since both organs are radiosensitive and are susceptible to deterministic somatic effects (i.e., cataracts and cancers).
- X-ray exams on children and adolescents should not be performed unless the benefit outweighs the risk, since their tissue is still developing.
- All equipment should be inspected routinely by a medical physicist to ensure optimal safety.
- Implement quality control and dose tracking practices with regular review of data to constantly strive for the best implementation of the ALARA principle.

Estimated General Patient Exposures [4]

- 1 mSv is the dose produced by exposure to 1 mGy.
- General public: 1 mSv per year, excluding medical tests derived from natural sources.
- Radiation workers—technologists and radiologists/support staff: 5 mSv.
    Dosimeters are required to be worn by all radiation personnel. These devices keep track of occupational dose and ensure that the working environment is safe. An external monitor is worn to monitor head and neck dose, and an internal device worn under the apron will monitor any dose penetrating the protective apron.
- Radiation sickness is induced at an exposure level of 500 mGy—single exposure.
- Cataracts: 500 mSv—cumulative dose.
- Human lethal dose (50% die in 30 days) = 5000 mGy—single dose.
- All interventional procedures are generally in the range of 1 mGy to 250 mGy.

Acknowledgments We would like to thank Prasaanthan Gopee-Ramanan and Sandra Reis for their contributions to this chapter (information given on first page of chapter).

References

1. Carlton RR, Adler AM, Balac V. Principles of radiographic imaging: an art and a science. 6th ed. Cengage Learning, Inc; 2018.
2. Dixon R, Whitlow C. The physical basis of diagnostic imaging. In: Chen M, Pope T, Ott D, editors. Basic radiology. 2nd ed. North Carolina: McGraw-Hill; 2010.
3. Government of Canada, H. C. H. E. A. C. P. S. B. Safety code 35: radiation protection in radiology—Large facilities; 2008. p. 1–88.
4. Kelsey CA, Heintz PH, Sandoval DJ, Chambers GD, Adolphi NL, Paffett KS. Radiation biology of medical imaging. Wiley, Incorporated; 2014.

Chapter 4
Common Equipment in Interventional Radiology

Anna Hwang and Jason Martin

Imaging Modalities

Fluoroscopy

Fluoroscopy is an imaging technique that uses X-rays to generate real-time images of patient anatomy and endovascular devices. Simply, a fluoroscope consists of an X-ray source and a fluorescent screen, in between which a patient is placed. Newer fluoroscopes utilize an X-ray image intensifier and a video camera, permitting the storage and playback of images. This modality is commonly used for guidewire and catheter manipulation.

Benefits include real-time imaging, portability, and the ability to save images for future reference and interpretation. Downsides include radiation exposure to the patient and the inability to clearly visualize visceral organs.

Fluoroscopy is best suited for most vascular and nonvascular interventional procedures [1].

A. Hwang (✉)
Michael G. DeGroote School of Medicine, McMaster University, Hamilton, ON, Canada
e-mail: anna.hwang@medportal.ca

J. Martin
Department of Medical Imaging, University of Toronto, Toronto, ON, Canada
e-mail: jason.martin@medportal.ca

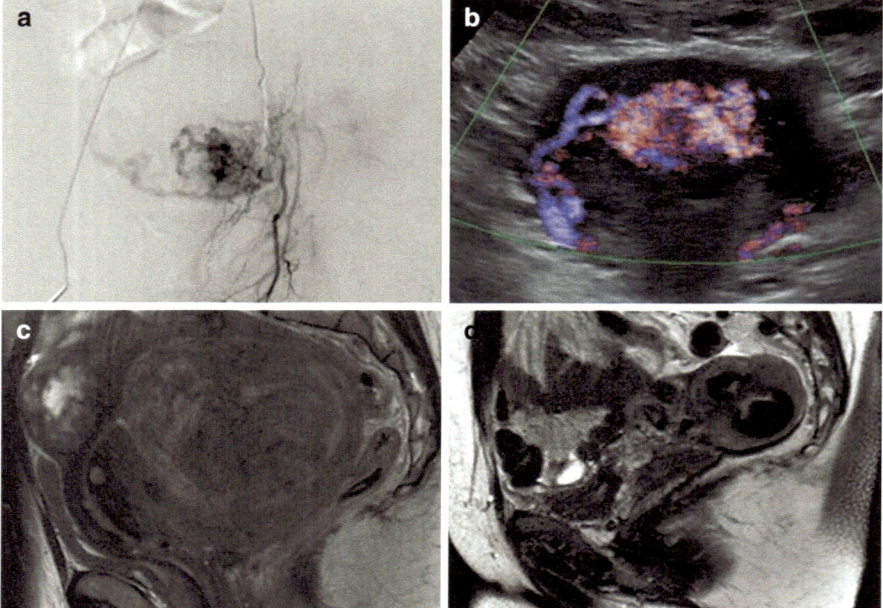

Fig. 4.1 Common modalities in interventional radiology (**a–d**). (**a**) Digital subtraction angiography of the uterine artery supplying a uterine fibroid. (**b**) Ultrasound with Doppler of uterine fibroid. (**c**) T2-weighted MRI of uterine fibroid. (**d**) T1-weighted MRI of uterine fibroid

Ultrasound

Ultrasound (U/S) utilizes sound waves to image internal organs or structures (Fig. 4.1). It is often used to achieve vascular access, to perform biopsies and drainage procedures.

Benefits include real-time guidance and manipulation, no radiation exposure to the patient, and lower cost. Downsides mainly surround the operator-dependent nature of the imaging.

Computed Tomography

Computed tomography (CT) uses X-rays to produce tomographic images (virtual slices) of areas of a scanned object, allowing one to see inside the body without cutting it open (Fig. 4.2). CT is used for solid organ biopsies and drainage procedures.

It is a useful adjunct for targets not visualized on ultrasound. Disadvantages include radiation dose, the visualization of the biopsy needle or the drainage catheter is not in real time, and the patient must be stable enough to be brought to the scanner and remain still.

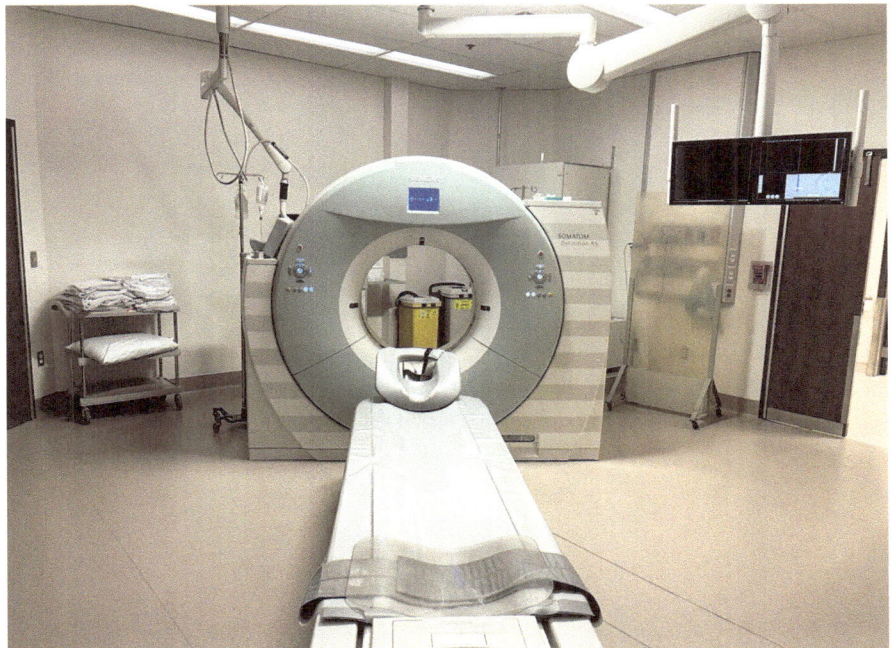

Fig. 4.2 Computed tomography (CT) scanner

Magnetic Resonance Imaging

Magnetic resonance imaging (MRI) offers excellent soft tissue contrast and high resolution of lesions. Advantages include no radiation dose and the avoidance of nephrotoxic iodinated contrast material. Downsides include the need for non-ferromagnetic devices, as well as patient stability during scanning and intervention.

Contrast

Contrast agents are used to improve the visibility of vessels and organs. Intravascular contrast is generally classified into ionic and non-ionic types. Ionic contrast media typically have higher osmolality and more side effects, while non-ionic contrast media typically have lower osmolality and fewer associated side effects.

Major complications from the use of iodinated contrast agents include anaphylactoid reactions and contrast-induced nephropathy. Anaphylactoid reactions can range from urticarial and itching to bronchospasm and laryngeal edema. Mild reactions can be managed with diphenhydramine, while IM epinephrine is more suitable for moderate to severe reactions. Blood pressure must be monitored closely, as hypotension may occur quite rapidly.

Contrast-induced nephropathy (CIN) is defined as either >25% increase or absolute 0.5 mg/dL increase in serum creatinine. *N*-Acetyl-cysteine does not appear to decrease rates of CIN. Adequate prehydration of patients is an intervention shown to reduce CIN rates in hospitalized patients [1].

Guidewires and Catheters

The basic apparatus for vascular intervention is the guidewire-catheter system. The catheter acts as a base of sorts, allowing the IR to maintain position within a vessel. The guidewire is used to explore further and, with its increased flexibility, take turns or round corners. They are not used in isolation, however. Catheters of different shapes may be used to direct a guidewire, and guidewires can be used alone to cross lesions, with the catheter following to maintain access beyond the lesion.

Guidewires

Guidewires (solid wires navigated within the vascular system) act as a lead point for catheters, allowing operators to traverse along a given vessel. They may differ in length, diameter, stiffness, and coating [1, 2].

Length

- Must be long enough to cover the distance both inside and outside the patient.
- Must also account for access well beyond the lesion, so that access across the lesion will not be lost intraoperatively.
- Guidewire lengths usually vary from 145 to 300 cm.

Diameter

- Vascular catheters are designed with a guidewire port of specific diameter.
- Most procedures are performed with O35 guidewires (0.035 in.).
- Small-vessel angioplasty (such as distal pedal) requires 0.018–0.014 in. guidewires.

Stiffness and Coating

- Most guidewires have a tightly wound steel core that contributes to body stiffness.
- A surrounding layer of flexible material prevents fracture during use.
- Teflon or silicone coatings are often used to reduce the friction coefficient and allow the operator smooth advancement within a vessel.

Tip Shape

- The shape of the guidewire tip often reveals the function of the guidewire.
- Floppy tip wires reduce the potential for vessel injury during access.
- Selective cannulation wires may be employed to traverse bends and curves and may be curved or angled to help the operator steer in a certain direction.

General Types of Guidewires

The three general types include starting, selective, and exchange guidewires:

- Starting guidewires are used for catheter introduction and some procedures.
- Selective guidewires are used to cannulate side branches or cross critical lesions.
- Exchange guidewires are stiffer and are used to secure position as devices are passed over the wire.

Catheters

The three general types of catheters are as follows (Fig. 4.3) [1, 2].

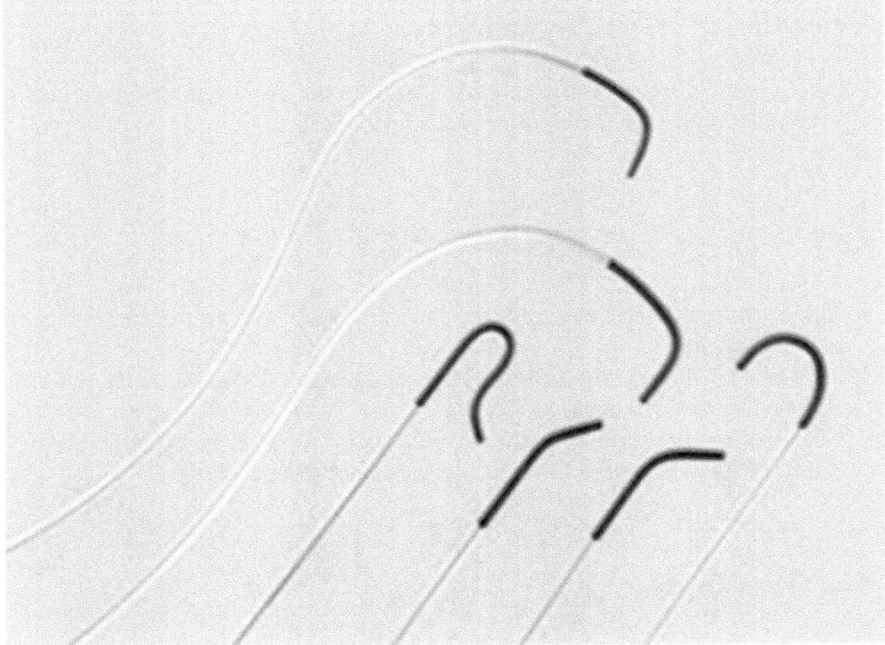

Fig. 4.3 A variety of differently shaped catheters for use in endovascular diagnosis and intervention

Vascular Dilator

- The simplest catheter, 12–15 cm with a single hole at the tip.
- Used to dilate the tract before insertion of catheter or sheaths, as well as secure vascular access or perform certain types of arteriography (usually femoral).

Exchange Catheter

- Generally straight and long.
- Used to exchange guidewires or for interval arteriography to monitor the progress of intervention.
- Provide multiple side holes for contrast administration. The catheter head is rounded to promote contrast blush.

Selective Catheter

- Come in a variety of head shapes.
- Used to direct a guidewire into a specific location.
- Some are designed for specific arteries (carotid, uterine, etc.).

Puncture Needles

Puncture needles are used to obtain passage from the skin to the target site before insertion of a guidewire, catheter, or other devices [1].

Type

- One-part needles have a sharp bevel and are used for simple procedures, such as arterial puncture.
- Two-part needles are used for deeper punctures and feature an inner stylet surrounded by an outer shaft.
- Sheathed needles have a plastic covering that stays in place after the needle is removed. These are used for many nonvascular procedures.

Size Considerations

- The higher the gauge, the smaller the lumen of the needle.

- Larger needles are easier to direct along the planned trajectory.
- Smaller needles are used for difficult punctures to minimize trauma.
- Many vascular procedures use a 19-gauge (G) needle, which fits a 0.035-inch guidewire.
- Nonvascular procedures often use larger needles, such as a 16G needle.
- The smallest puncture needle used in most departments is 21 G, which fits a 0.018-inch guidewire.

Biopsy Needles

Biopsy needles are used to obtain a sample for diagnosis. Two main types of biopsy needles include aspiration and core biopsy needles [1].

Aspiration Needle

- Used to sample a few cells for analysis.
- 21G needles are commonly used, but size can range from 20 to 25G.
- The needle is inserted into the lesion under ultrasound guidance, and suction is applied with a syringe.
- Gentle suction is maintained as the needle is withdrawn.
- The contents of the needle are ejected using an air-filled syringe.

Cutting Biopsy Needle

- Used to obtain larger samples for histological study.
- 18G needles are commonly used, but size can range from 14 to 20G.
- Has an inner stylet with an outer cutting shaft.
- Most IR departments use automatic, spring-loaded devices that advance the outer cutting shaft upon the push of a button.
- The shortest possible needle should be used to minimize trauma while still obtaining a reliable sample.

Stents

Stents provide structural support to keep vessels patent. A stent consists of a metal latticework that is compressed prior to insertion, but then expands to a much larger diameter. Stents can be either self-expanding or balloon expandable. A self-expanding stent is held in place by an outer sheath as it is passed along the delivery catheter. The sheath is retracted once the target site is reached, causing the stent to expand. Most balloon expandable stents come already mounted on a balloon catheter [1].

References

1. Kessel D, Robertson I. Interventional radiology: a survival guide. 4th ed. Philadelphia: Elsevier; 2017.
2. Schneider PA. Endovascular skills—guidewire and catheter skills for endovascular surgery. 2nd ed. New York: Marcel Dekker; 2003.

Chapter 5
Medications Used in Interventional Radiology

Lazar Milovanovic and Ashis Bagchee-Clark

Pre-procedural Medications

Anticoagulation

Anticoagulation is an important consideration in pre-procedural assessment of patients. Many interventional procedures, especially those requiring vascular access, may lead to increased rates of hemorrhage if the coagulation status of the patient is not managed appropriately. The difficulty arises when considering the need to balance an increased bleeding risk during and after an IR procedure with thromboembolic risk if anticoagulants are to be stopped [1].

Many patients presenting for interventional radiological procedures will be on short- or long-term anticoagulation, as well as antiplatelet medications [1]. The management of coagulation status is challenging due to the lack of strong evidence for approaches to patients with abnormal coagulation test values [1]. Some of the recommendations for interventional radiologists to manage coagulation status are based on extrapolation of surgical data [1]. When planning interventional procedures, there are many factors to consider including patient characteristics, procedure type, procedure urgency, and postprocedural management strategies. A summary of the common interventional radiology procedures with low and high bleeding risk is presented in Table 5.1 [1]. The management for patients undergoing these procedures is presented in Table 5.2 [1].

Two important groups of patients on anticoagulation agents presenting for interventional procedures are inpatients with prophylactic anticoagulation to prevent

L. Milovanovic · A. Bagchee-Clark (✉)
Michael G. DeGroote School of Medicine, McMaster University, Hamilton, ON, Canada
e-mail: lazar.milovanovic@medportal.ca; ashis.bagcheeclark@medportal.ca

Table 5.1 Categorization of procedures by bleeding risk [1]

Procedures with low bleeding risk	Procedures with high bleeding risk
• Catheter exchanges (gastrostomy, biliary, nephrostomy, abscess, including gastrostomy/ gastrojejunostomy conversions) • Diagnostic arteriography and arterial interventions: peripheral, sheath <6 F, embolotherapy • Diagnostic venography and select venous interventions: pelvis and extremities • Dialysis access interventions • Facet joint injections and medial branch nerve blocks (thoracic and lumbar spine) • IVC filter placement and removal • Lumbar puncture • Nontunneled chest tube placement for pleural effusion • Nontunneled venous access and removal (including PICC placement) • Paracentesis • Peripheral nerve blocks, joint, and musculoskeletal injections • Sacroiliac joint injection and sacral lateral branch blocks • Superficial abscess drainage or biopsy (palpable lesion, lymph node, soft tissue, breast, thyroid, superficial bone, e.g., extremities and bone marrow aspiration) • Thoracentesis • Transjugular liver biopsy • Trigger point injections including piriformis • Tunneled drainage catheter placement • Tunneled venous catheter placement/removal (including ports)	• Ablations: solid organs, bone, soft tissue, lung • Arterial interventions: > 7-F sheath, aortic, pelvic, mesenteric, CNS • Biliary interventions (including cholecystostomy tube placement) • Catheter-directed thrombolysis (DVT, PE, portal vein) • Deep abscess drainage (e.g., lung parenchyma, abdominal, pelvic, retroperitoneal) • Deep nonorgan biopsies (e.g., spine, soft tissue in intra-abdominal, retroperitoneal, pelvic compartments) • Gastrostomy/gastrojejunostomy placement • IVC filter removal complex • Portal vein interventions • Solid organ biopsies • Spine procedures with risk of spinal or epidural hematoma (e.g., kyphoplasty, vertebroplasty, epidural injections, facet blocks cervical spine) • Transjugular intrahepatic portosystemic shunt • Urinary tract interventions (including nephrostomy tube placement, ureteral dilation, stone removal) • Venous interventions: intrathoracic and CNS interventions

IVC inferior vena cava, *PICC* peripherally inserted central catheter

Table 5.2 Procedure bleeding risk, appropriate testing, and consensus management [1]

Procedure bleeding risk	Pre-procedure lab testing	Management
Low risk	• PT/INR: not routinely recommended • Platelet count/ hemoglobin: not routinely recommended	• INR: correct to within range of ≤2.0–3.0 • Platelets: transfuse if <20 × 10^9/L • UFH and LMWH: do not withhold • Warfarin: target INR ≤3.0; consider bridging for high thrombosis risk cases • Apixaban: do not withhold • Clopidogrel and aspirin: do not withhold
High risk	• PT/INR: routinely recommended • Platelet count/ hemoglobin: routinely recommended	• INR: correct to within range of ≤1.5–1.8 • Platelets: transfuse if <50 × 10^9/L • UFH: withhold IV heparin for 4–6 h before procedure; check aPTT or anti-Xa level; for BID or TID dosing of SC heparin, procedure may be performed 6 h after last dose

Table 5.2 (continued)

Procedure bleeding risk	Pre-procedure lab testing	Management
		• LMWH: enoxaparin, withhold 1 dose if prophylactic dose is used; withhold 2 doses or 24 h before procedure if therapeutic dose is used; dalteparin, withhold 1 dose before procedure • Warfarin: withhold 5 d until target INR ≤1.8; consider bridging for high thrombosis risk cases; if STAT or emergent, use reversal agent • Apixaban: withhold 4 doses (CrCl ≥50 mL/min) or 6 doses (CrCl <30–50 mL/min); if procedure is STAT or emergent, use reversal agent (andexanet alfa); consider checking anti-Xa activity or apixaban level especially with impaired renal function • Clopidogrel/aspirin: withhold 3–5 days before the procedure

deep vein thrombosis and patients with atrial fibrillation on anticoagulation to reduce risk of stroke. Greater thromboembolic risk is seen in patients with past history of a thromboembolic event, cancer, and valvular heart disease [1].

Prophylactic Antibiotics

Different procedures in interventional radiology have varying levels of risk of infection [2, 3]:

- Clean procedures—spaces potentially containing bacteria (gastrointestinal, biliary, genitourinary, respiratory tracts, infected or inflamed tissue) are avoided.
- Clean-contaminated procedures—if the procedure leads to entering a space containing bacteria that is not inflamed.
- Contaminated procedures—space containing inflammation is entered.
- Dirty procedures—pus and free spillage of contaminated material occur.

Antibiotic prophylaxis recommended in interventional radiological procedures not classified as clean. The selection of antibiotic depends on procedure, organ system, locoregional sensitivities, and costs (Table 5.3). Timing and duration of prophylactic antibiotic administration is based on surgical literature data, and a single pre-procedural dose of the appropriate antimicrobial agent is recommended within 1 h of commencement of most procedures [4].

Table 5.3 Recommended antibiotic prophylaxis for interventional radiology procedures

Procedure	Procedure type	Common organisms	Routine prophylaxis
Vascular interventions: Angiography, angioplasty, atherectomy, thrombolysis, stent placement, arterial closure device placement	Clean	Skin flora	Not recommended
Endograft placement (aortic, peripheral)	Clean	Skin flora	Cefazolin IV; alt: Vancomycin or clindamycin if penicillin allergy
Superficial venous insufficiency treatment (lower extremity)	Clean	Skin flora	Not recommended
IVC filter placement	Clean	None	Not recommended
Chemoembolization and embolization	Clean or clean contaminated	*S. aureus*, *Streptococcus* species, *Corynebacterium* species	No consensus first-choice antibiotic; hepatic chemoembo, ampicillin/sulbactam IV, cefazolin and metronidazole, ampicillin IV, and gentamicin; embolization or chemoembo, ceftriaxone IV
Uterine artery embolization	Clean or clean contaminated	Skin flora, *Streptococcus* species, *E. coli*	No consensus first choice; cefazolin IV, clindamycin IV plus gentamicin; ampicillin IV; ampicillin/sulbactam IV; vancomycin if penicillin allergy
Transjugular intrahepatic portosystemic shunt (TIPS) creation	Clean or clean contaminated	Skin flora, *Corynebacterium* species, biliary pathogens, enteric Gram-negative rods, anaerobes, *Enterococcus* species	No consensus first choice; ceftriaxone IV; ampicillin/sulbactam IV; if penicillin allergic: Vancomycin or clindamycin or aminoglycoside
Percutaneous gastrostomy and gastrojejunostomy placement	Clean contaminated	Skin flora, *Corynebacterium* species	Recommended for pull technique, no consensus for push technique; cefazolin IV for pull technique is first choice
Subcutaneous venous access ports, immunocompetent patients	Clean	None	None
Subcutaneous venous access ports, immunocompromised patients	Clean	*Staphylococcus*	Cefazolin

Table 5.3 (continued)

Procedure	Procedure type	Common organisms	Routine prophylaxis
Transhepatic cholangiography and percutaneous biliary drainage; no signs of biliary infection, no history of surgery or instrumentation	Clean or clean contaminated	*Klebsiella, Enterobacter, E. coli*	Ceftriaxone
Transhepatic cholangiography and percutaneous biliary drainage; prior bilioenteric anastomosis or instrumentation	Clean or clean contaminated	*Klebsiella, Enterobacter, E. coli*	Piperacillin–tazobactam or ticarcillin–clavulanic acid or ampicillin/ sulbactam
Biliary tube replacement (clean contaminated)	Clean contaminated	*Klebsiella, Enterobacter, E. coli*	Ceftriaxone or piperacillin–tazobactam or ticarcillin–clavulanic acid or ampicillin/ sulbactam
Radiofrequency ablation of liver tumor	Clean contaminated	*Klebsiella, Enterobacter, E. coli*	Ceftriaxone or piperacillin–tazobactam or ticarcillin–clavulanic acid or ampicillin/ sulbactam
Antegrade pyelography and percutaneous nephrostomy	Clean or clean contaminated	None	Cefazolin
Nephrostomy tube change	Clean contaminated	*E. coli, P. mirabilis, Enterococcus, Pseudomonas*	None
Abdominal fluid aspiration of uninfected ascites, lymphocele, or simple hepatic or renal cyst	Clean	None	None

Adapted from [3, 4]
Alt alternate, skin flora *S. aureus* and *S. epidermidis*

When a patient requires procedures with instrumentation and drainage of obstructed infected collection or system (biliary, kidney obstruction, liver abscess), the risk of post-procedural bacteremia is significantly higher until drainage is complete [3, 5]; antibiotic treatment should last from immediately prior to procedure until drainage is complete [4]. If a procedure lasts longer than 2 h, an additional dose of antibiotic can be considered [4]. Table 5.4 presents a summary of the potential risk factors for infective endocarditis in patients undergoing interventional procedures and whether antibiotic prophylaxis is recommended [3, 5].

Table 5.4 Risk factors for bacterial endocarditis—indications for antibiotic prophylaxis

Condition	Details	Antibiotic prophylaxis
Prosthetic cardiac valves	Bioprosthetic or homograft	Required
Previous bacterial endocarditis	With or without heart disease	Required
Congenital cardiac malformations	Not isolated secundum atrial septal defect	Required
Surgically constructed systemic pulmonary shunts or conduits		Required
Acquired valvular dysfunction, including rheumatic	Pre- and post-valvular surgery	Required
Hypertrophic cardiomyopathy		Required
Mitral valve prolapse	With valvular regurgitation and/or thickened leaflets	Required
Surgical repair of ASD, VSD, or PDA	Without residual beyond 6 months	Not required
Previous coronary artery bypass graft surgery		Not required
Mitral valve prolapse	Without valvular regurgitation	Not required
Heart murmurs	Physiologic, functional, or innocent	Not required
Previous Kawasaki disease	Without valvular dysfunction	Not required
Previous rheumatic fever	Without valvular dysfunction	Not required
Cardiac pacemakers and implanted defibrillators		Not required

Adapted from [3, 5]

X-Ray Contrast Media

Contrast media is used throughout diagnostic imaging for both diagnostic and image guidance purposes during interventional procedures in order to increase the difference in contrast between tissues and help differentiate structures as well as identify vasculature. Contrast is differentiated by the type of study to be completed: magnetic resonance imaging (MRI) contrast has different properties than X-ray contrast, which is used in computed tomography (CT), plain radiography, and fluoroscopy.

X-ray contrast can be differentiated into positive and negative contrast agents depending on their composition. Positive contrast media agents cause increased attenuation of X-rays compared to the surrounding patient tissue and appear dark under fluoroscopy; these agents contain iodine. Negative contrast media agents cause less attenuation of X-rays than the surrounding patient tissue and appear lighter under fluoroscopy; the only negative contrast available is carbon dioxide gas. Iodinated (iodine-containing) positive contrast agents can be further subdivided into ionic and nonionic depending on the specific molecular structure of the contrast agent to be used (Table 5.5) [6].

Table 5.5 Overview of iodinated contrast agents [6]

Type	Generation	Alternative names	Generic name
Iodinated ionic	First generation	High-osmolar contrast media (HOCM)	• Diatrizoate meglumine • Diatrizoate sodium • Diatrizoate meglumine and diatrizoate sodium mixture
Iodinated nonionic	Second generation	Low-osmolar contrast media (LOCM)	• Iohexol • Iopamidol • Iopromide • Ioversol
Iodinated nonionic iso-osmolar	Third generation	N/A	• Iodixanol

Iodinated Contrast Complications and Side Effects

There are multiple risk factors predisposing patients to contrast reactions including:

- Infants and patients over the age of 60
- Female gender
- Underlying asthma, heart disease, dehydration, renal disease, or diabetes
- Hematologic conditions including myeloma, sickle cell disease, or polycythemia
- Use of nonsteroidal anti-inflammatory drugs (NSAIDs), interleukin-2 (IL-2) chemotherapy, beta-blockers, or biguanides (metformin, glyburide, Glucophage, Metaglip)
- Contrast-related factors including large quantities of iodine (>20 mg), fast injection rate, intra-arterial injection, and history of contrast reactions [7]

Mild complications may include headache, nausea and/or vomiting, skin flushing, pruritus, mild skin rash, or hives.

Moderate complications may include arrhythmias, hypotension or hypertension, dyspnea or difficulty breathing, wheezing, and severe skin rash or hives.

Severe reactions may include cardiac arrest, anaphylaxis, difficulty breathing, convulsions, air embolism, and severe hypotension.

Contrast media-induced nephropathy is defined as an increase in the serum creatinine by more than 0.5 mg/dL (44.2 μ[mu]mol/L) or an increase of more than 50% above baseline over a period of 1–3 days postinjection [7].

Peri- and Intra-procedural Medications

Vasoconstrictors

Vasoconstrictors [8] are primarily used for acute gastroenterological bleeding. The main vasoconstrictor utilized is vasopressin. Vasopressin (exogenous form of antidiuretic hormone, ADH) promotes contraction of vascular smooth muscle of the small arterioles, capillaries, and small venules [9]. Vasopressin infusion is indicated in GI bleed cases where embolization is contraindicated or cannot be performed such as in diffuse mucosal bleeding. The efficacy of vasopressin is reduced in patients with atherosclerosis due to reduced constriction of arterioles in the presence of plaques.

Common adverse reactions to vasopressin may include headache, diaphoresis, nausea and vomiting, and abdominal cramps [9]. Complications of vasopressin may include ischemic and cardiovascular effects such as bowel infarction and peripheral vascular ischemia as well as hypertension, arrhythmias, and myocardial infarction, respectively [9]. Delayed complications may occur secondary to antidiuretic effects such as electrolyte instability, hypertension, and oliguria [9].

Vasodilators

Vasodilators [8] are used in the prevention or management of arterial spasm. They are also used to increase blood flow in distal arteries in order to enhance visualization.

Nitroglycerine (NG) is a short-acting vasodilator that relaxes vascular smooth muscle cells. It takes effect instantaneously, and the total duration varies based on dose, but is usually several minutes [9].

Verapamil is a calcium channel blocker that relaxes smooth muscle cells while also decreasing the rate of conduction of electrical signals through the AV node, depressing the heart rate [9]. Verapamil has a longer duration of action and is considered more potent than NG; however, NG is preferred for catheter-induced vasospasm prevention and treatment [9].

During administration of vasodilators, it is important to carefully monitor the blood pressure of the patient. Complications may include systemic hypotension, headache, tachycardia, and nausea and vomiting. Contraindications for vasodilators include elevated intracranial pressure, constrictive pericarditis, pericardial tamponade, and previous hypersensitivity reaction.

Anxiolytic

An anxiolytic can be used shortly prior to the procedure. The principal function of an anxiolytic is typically to reduce patient anxiety; anxiolytics such as diazepam have additional practical usage in interventional radiology procedures as an amnestic, anticonvulsant, and muscle relaxant [1].

An important consideration when using anxiolytics is the synergistic effect they often possess with many medications used in sedation. As such, one should take special care to adjust the dose of a sedative if an anxiolytic is to be used in combination [1].

Local Analgesics

Local anesthetics are injected into the tissues prior to intervention in order to minimize patient discomfort and pain at the local access site.

Lidocaine (trade name: Xylocaine) is the most common analgesic agent encountered in the interventional suite and is available as both a topical and an injectable [1]. When used as an injectable, it is administered in various solutions from 0.5% to 5% [1]. It has a rapid onset of effect of less than 5 min and lasts approximately 1 h. Lidocaine is arrhythmogenic if injected into the vasculature or delivered by IV, so care must be taken to avoid arteries and veins when injecting it locally. In individuals who are adverse to needles, an emulsion of 2.5% lidocaine and 2.5% prilocaine applied an hour prior to the procedure can supply effective analgesia [10].

Sedatives

For interventional radiology procedures, sedation and analgesia should allow purposeful response to verbal or tactile stimulation with no airway intervention required; adequate spontaneous ventilation and cardiovascular function are usually maintained.

There are many different choices for achieving this level of sedation, and selection of appropriate medication depends on the patient, the type of procedure, and the preference of the interventional radiologist. Medications, largely opioids and benzodiazepines, which can achieve moderate sedation are shown in Table 5.6 [11].

Table 5.6 Medications used in moderate sedation

Medication	Class	Dose	Time to onset (min)	Duration	Pregnancy category
Midazolam	Benzodiazepine	< 1.0 mg IV	1–3	1 h	D
Diazepam	Benzodiazepine	1.0–2.0 mg IV	2–3	6 h	D
Lorazepam	Benzodiazepine	2.0 mg P.O.	Up to 60–90	10–20 h	D
Morphine	Opioid	2.0 mg IV	10	4 h	C
Fentanyl	Opioid	25 µg IV	2–3	30–60 min	C
Hydromorphone	Opioid	1.0 mg IV; use smallest effective dose	10	4–5 h	C
Meperidine		10–25 mg IV	5–15	2–4 h	C
Ketorolac	NSAID	30–60 mg IM			C (first and second trimesters), D (third trimester)

(continued)

Table 5.6 (continued)

Medication	Class	Dose	Time to onset (min)	Duration	Pregnancy category
Flumazenil	Benzodiazepine antagonist	200 µg IV per minute (up to 1 mg)	1	30–60 min	C
Naloxone	Opioid reversal agent	0.1–0.3 mg q 30–60 s	Rapid	20–30 min	C

Adapted from [11]
NSAID nonsteroidal anti-inflammatory drug

Opioids and benzodiazepines have synergistic effects and side effects; consequently, when used in combination, smaller doses of both should be utilized to achieve adequate sedation, with the opioid administered first to achieve adequate analgesia prior to any elicited pain [1]. Owing to rapid onset, short duration of action, and ease in successful titration, fentanyl and midazolam are becoming increasingly used versus the historically more common morphine and diazepam [1].

Bowel Antiperistalsis Agents

Buscopan is an antispasmodic agent used to reduce peristalsis and relieve smooth muscle spasms in the stomach, intestines, bladder, and urethra. It can be used to optimize radiographic visualization of the GI tract and facilitate procedures involving the GI tract by reducing bowel tone and spasm [12]. Buscopan can be administered via intravenous or oral methods.

Glucagon inhibits GI motility, leading to optimization of radiographic visualization of the GI tract, and facilitates procedures involving the GI tract by reducing bowel tone and spasm [9]. Glucagon must be administered by IV or intramuscular injection due to complete breakdown of the compound by gastrointestinal enzymes when given orally [8].

Post-procedural Medications

Analgesics

Common post-procedural analgesics used by interventional radiologists include ketorolac, oxycodone, hydromorphone, and acetaminophen [8, 9, 13]:

- Ketorolac (Toradol)—an NSAID and reversible COX inhibitor administered intravenously or by oral route with an onset of action of 20 min and duration of action of 4–6 h.

- Oxycodone (OxyContin)—an opioid agonist with a 30 min onset of action and 3–4 h duration of action.
- Acetaminophen (Tylenol)—a centrally acting analgesic and antipyretic with a 20–45 min onset of action and 4–6 h duration of action. Acetaminophen can be hepatotoxic and should not be used in patients with liver dysfunction.
- Hydromorphone (Dilaudid)—an opioid agonist used to treat moderate to severe pain with an onset of action of 15 min (parenterally) and 30 min (orally) and a duration of more than 5 h.

Antimicrobial Therapy

There are many factors that affect whether a patient requires antimicrobial therapy in the post-procedural setting including procedure type, procedure duration, procedure complications, and patient characteristics including immune status. Decisions on post-procedure antimicrobial therapy are usually made with input from the interventional radiologist and the most responsible physician as well as guidance from infectious disease physicians in specific situations.

Antiemetics

Antiemetics are used for the management of nausea and vomiting and are particularly important for patients undergoing oncologic or palliative procedures [13]. Nausea and vomiting can also occur commonly as part of post-embolic syndrome:

- Ondansetron—a selective serotonin 5HT3 receptor antagonist commonly given orally or intravenously, used for post-procedure prophylaxis in adults. It is often used for patients undergoing chemotherapy or radiotherapy but also indicated as an antiemetic for patients post-surgery [9].
- Promethazine—a phenothiazine utilized for the antihistamine (H1)-blocking characteristics of the compound leading to antiemetic and anti-motion properties on administration to patients [9]. Promethazine has some sedative effects and can be used along with analgesics during patient sedation [9].
- Scopolamine—an acetylcholine muscarinic receptor antagonist that has been shown to be useful in the treatment of nausea and vomiting secondary to motion sickness due to action on the vestibular pathways between the inner ear and brainstem [9].

Anticoagulation

There are only some procedures that require interruption of anticoagulation and antiplatelet therapy, as previously described in Table 5.2. In cases where anticoagulation is withheld, anticoagulation and antiplatelet therapy is usually reinitiated immediately post-procedure. High-risk patients for thrombosis can have their time off anticoagulation minimized by transitioning the patient to agents such as heparin as inpatients [1]. A summary of the different anticoagulation and antiplatelet therapies, monitoring procedures, reversal agents, and recommended periprocedural administration protocols is presented in Table 5.7 [2, 14].

In certain cases with increased risk of bleeding post-procedure, the decision to hold anticoagulation and antiplatelet therapy is made by the interventional radiologist along with input from the most responsible physician.

Table 5.7 Periprocedural management of anticoagulants

Agent	Medication class	Lab monitoring	Reversal agent	Last dose—procedure interval
Warfarin	Vitamin K agonist	INR	Vitamin K with or without FFP; 3- or 4-factor PCCs	INR dependent, usually 1–8 days
Unfractionated heparin	Heparins	aPTT	Protamine sulfate	IV: 2–6 h; subcut: 12–24 h
LMWH	Heparins	None regularly—Anti-factor Xa antibody levels in select pts	Protamine sulfate (results in partial reversal only)	Low or moderate risk: 1 dose High risk: 24 h
Fondaparinux	Heparins	None	None—May use recombinant factor VIIa in high-risk pts. with major bleed	36–48 h
Dabigatran	Direct thrombin inhibitor	None—aPTT or thrombin time for substantial residual effect	None—Consider factor VIII inhibitor bypass activity or recombinant VIIa, hemodialysis	CrCl: ≥50 mL/min—1–2 days CrCl: <50 mL/min—3–5 days
Rivaroxaban	Direct factor Xa inhibitor	None—Prothrombin time or anti-factor Xa antibody to rule out substantial residual effect	None—Consider PCCs	Normal renal function: ≥1 day CrCl: 60–90 mL/min—2 days CrCl: 30–59 mL/min—3 days CrCl: 15–29 mL/min—4 days
Apixaban	Direct factor Xa inhibitor	None—Anti-factor Xa antibody to rule out substantial residual effect	None—Consider charcoal hemoperfusion or PCCs	CrCl: ≥60 mL/min—1–2 days CrCl: 50–59 mL/min—3 days CrCl: <30–49 mL/min—5 days

Table 5.7 (continued)

Agent	Medication class	Lab monitoring	Reversal agent	Last dose—procedure interval
Desirudin	Direct thrombin inhibitor	aPTT, thrombin time, ecarin clotting time—Normal value rules out clinically relevant residual effect	None	2 h
Aspirin	Antiplatelet agent	None—Consider platelet function tests	Platelet transfusion	Low or moderate risk: None High risk: 5 days
Thienopyridine agents (clopidogrel, ticlopidine, prasugrel, ticagrelor)	Antiplatelet agents—ADP receptor/P2Y12 inhibitor	None—Consider platelet function tests	Consider platelet transfusion (limited efficacy)	Clopidogrel/ticagrelor—5 days Prasugrel—7 days Ticlopidine—10–14 days

Adapted from [2, 14]
FFP fresh frozen plasma, *PCC* prothrombin complex concentrate, *LMWH* low molecular weight heparin, *CrCl* creatinine clearance

Summary

In the pre-procedural setting, medications play a key role in minimizing patient risk of bleeding and infection; it is important to evaluate the procedure and patient for possible risk factors for bleeding and infection and adjust pre-procedural medication accordingly.

Intra-procedural medications help sedate and anesthetize patients, alter vascular muscle tone, and reduce peristalsis for gastric interventions and detailed imaging.

Post-procedural medications are helpful in managing pain, nausea and vomiting, bleeding risk, and infection. Knowledge of the procedure outcome, complications, patient factors, and future management are important factors affecting decisions for post-procedural medications.

References

1. Patel IJ, Rahim S, Davidson JC, Hanks SE, Tam AL, Walker TG, Wilkins LR, Sarode R, Weinberg I. Society of Interventional Radiology consensus guidelines for the periprocedural management of thrombotic and bleeding risk in patients undergoing percutaneous image-guided interventions—part II: recommendations: endorsed by the Canadian Association for Interventional Radiology and the Cardiovascular and Interventional Radiological Society of Europe. J Vasc Interv Radiol. 2019;30(8):1168–84.

2. Patel IJ, Davidson JC, Nikolic B, et al. Consensus guidelines for periprocedural management of coagulation status and hemostasis risk in percutaneous image-guided interventions. J Vasc Interv Radiol. 2012;23:727–36.

3. Zarrinpar A, Kerlan RK Jr. A guide to antibiotics for the interventional radiologist. Semin Intervent Radiol. 2005;22(2):69–79.

4. Venkatesan AM, Kundu S, Sacks D, et al. Practice guidelines for adult antibiotic prophylaxis during vascular and interventional radiology procedures. J Vasc Interv Radiol. 2010;21:1611–30.

5. Dajani AS, Taubert KA, Wilson W, et al. Prevention of bacterial endocarditis. Recommendations by the American Heart Association. JAMA. 1997;277(22):1794–801.

6. Widmark JM. Imaging-related medications: a class overview. Proc (Bayl Univ Med Cent). 2007;20(4):408–17.

7. Singh J, Daftary A. Iodinated contrast media and their adverse reactions. J Nucl Med Technol. 2008;36(2):69–74.

8. Oppenheimer J, Ray CE Jr, Kondo KL. Miscellaneous pharmaceutical agents in interventional radiology. Semin Intervent Radiol. 2010;27(4):422–30.

9. Interventional Radiology Drugs on the Web. www.irdrugs.com/Class/class_sedation.html. Accessed 11 Jun 2014.

10. Johnson S. Sedation and analgesia in the performance of interventional procedures. Semin Interv Radiol. 2010;27:368–73.

11. Olsen JW, Barger RL Jr, Doshi SK. Moderate sedation: what radiologists need to know. AJR Am J Roentgenol. 2013;201:941–6.

12. Marti-Bonmati L, Graells M, Ronchera-Oms CL. Reduction of peristaltic artifacts on magnetic resonance imaging of the abdomen: a comparative evaluation of three drugs. Abdom Imaging. 1996;21(4):309–13.

13. Prescription drug information, interactions & side effects. www.drugs.com. Accessed 11 Jun 2014.

14. Baron TH, Kamath PS, McBane RD. Management of antithrombotic therapy in patients undergoing invasive procedures. N Engl J Med. 2013;368(22):2113–24.

Chapter 6
Interventional Radiology Outpatient Clinics

Ibrahim Mohammad Nadeem, Ruqqiyah Rana, and Lazar Milovanovic

Background

IRs have a unique skill set within the healthcare field and contribute with a specific role in patient care. Over the past four decades, there has been a shift in recognizing the role of IRs as clinicians and not just proceduralists. The practice of IR has evolved into one that requires longitudinal care of the patient—including before, during, and after interventions. Therefore, the primary goal of an outpatient IR clinic is to increase direct interaction with patients, provide counseling regarding disease and the available therapeutic options, and create and implement management plans. Unlike diagnostic radiologists, interventionalists require clinic time, clinic space, and additional procedure time to optimize their practice.

I. M. Nadeem (✉)
Department of Radiology, Faculty of Health Sciences, McMaster University,
Hamilton, ON, Canada
e-mail: ibrahim.nadeem@medportal.ca

R. Rana
Michael G. DeGroote School of Medicine, McMaster University, Hamilton, ON, Canada
e-mail: ruqqiyah.rana@medportal.ca

L. Milovanovic
Department of Critical Care Medicine, Faculty of Medicine and Dentistry, University of
Alberta, Edmonton, AB, Canada
e-mail: lazar.milovanovic@medportal.ca

S. Athreya, M. Albahhar (eds.), *Demystifying Interventional Radiology*,
https://doi.org/10.1007/978-3-031-12023-7_6

Infrastructure Requirements

Physical Space

The standard domains of diagnostic radiology, including hospital radiology departments and outpatient imaging centers, are not designed for the non-imaging patient consultations required for an IR practice. Physical consult space is required where the interventionalist can interview and examine patients in private [1].

Support Staff

This varies depending on the radiology practice and can involve nurse practitioners, physician assistants, nurses, clinical nurse specialists, and nonclinical support staff including receptionists and administrative assistants [1].

Appointment Scheduling

In addition to procedural requests from other inpatient departments, appropriate organization and scheduling of appointments is a key component to ensuring an outpatient IR practice thrives [1].

Responsibilities of Interventional Radiologists in Clinical Practice

In order to assist IRs in taking on the roles of clinician and care provider, the American College of Radiology has developed practice guidelines for IR practices, within which they have defined the responsibilities of IRs to be the following [2, 3]:

1. Interventional clinicians will serve as primary consultants for a particular disease and will accept referrals for therapeutic assessment for this disease and conduct patient consultations prior to and after the planned or elective intervention [2].
2. Interventional clinicians will engage with referred patients to perform diagnostic clarification, explore various therapeutic options, and provide the intervention requested by the patient [2].
3. Interventional clinicians will assume a strong role in treatment planning by developing and implementing treatment plans without participation of other

specialists, except in cases where multidisciplinary collaboration assists in patient care [2].
4. Interventional clinicians will accept clinical duties in the hospital and admit patients to the interventional service in order to manage post-procedural complications and recovery [2].
5. Interventional clinicians will engage in longitudinal patient care beyond the peri-procedural period [2].

Advantages to Strong Clinical Practices

There are many advantages to developing a strong outpatient clinical practice that serves to improve the patient experience, the practice parameters of the IR, and the future potential of the field of IR.

Advantages include:

- Opportunity to expand the referral base for IRs from community physicians rather than exclusively through other specialists [4, 5].
- The patient is provided multiple opportunities to ask questions regarding the disease, procedure, and possible complications throughout the consultation process [4, 5].
- The interventionalist is able to cultivate a stronger relationship with referring surgical and medical clinicians, developing a mutually beneficial referral process in order to optimize patient care [4, 5].
- Increased contact and development of a stronger clinician-patient relationship with the goal to increase patient and physician satisfaction [6].
- Strong clinical practices provide the opportunity for interventional clinicians to engage in more consistent follow-up, enabling the clinician to provide high-quality longitudinal care for their patients [6].

Pre-procedural Clinic and Initial Consults

Patients are referred from specialists or community physicians for a particular condition for which percutaneous IR procedures can provide therapeutic management. Studies have shown that the number of referrals to outpatient IR clinics has increased by at least 130% over the last decade [7]. The most common clinic referrals are for uterine fibroid (leiomyoma) embolization, tumor ablation, kyphoplasty and vertebroplasty, saphenous vein ablation, lower extremity arterial stents, renal artery stents, and transjugular intrahepatic portosystemic shunt (TIPS) [8] (Table 6.1).

A history and physical exam are conducted on the patient by IRs, who evaluates or orders appropriate high-quality planning imaging. The patient's clinical status

Table 6.1 Pre- and post-procedural tests and follow-up interval for common interventional radiology procedures

Procedure	Pre-procedural visit tests and imaging	Routine post-procedural visits	
		Timing	Imaging
Uterine fibroid embolization	Pre- and postcontrast MRI	2 weeks, 6 months	Pre- and postcontrast MRI
Tumor ablation (radiofrequency, chemoembolization, radioembolization)	Pre- and postcontrast CT scan, US for RFA patients	1 month, every 3 months following	Pre- and postcontrast CT scan at each visit
Kyphoplasty and vertebroplasty	Plain films, MRI spine	1 month	None—Unless clinically indicated
Saphenous vein ablation	Lower extremity US	1 month	Lower extremity US
Lower extremity arterial stents	Pulse volume recording, magnetic resonance angiography	1 month, 4 months, every 6 months following	PVR at each visit
Renal artery stents	CTA or MRA	1 month, every 6 months following	US at each visit
TIPS	US or CT	2 weeks, every 3 months for 1 year, every 6 months following	US at each visit

Adapted from [8]

TIPS transjugular intrahepatic portosystemic shunt, *US* ultrasound, *CT* computed tomography, *CTA* computed tomography angiography, *MRA* magnetic resonance angiography, *MRI* magnetic resonance imaging

and burden of disease are evaluated to triage the disease severity and procedure. The interventionalist explains therapeutic options, benefits, possible complications, and alternatives to the patient, and patients are provided with an opportunity to ask questions regarding procedure and management options.

Post-procedural Clinic and Follow-Up

Following the procedure, the interventionalist assesses wound healing and any procedural complications, especially if ionizing radiation was utilized. Routine follow-up imaging reassesses the pathologic status. In addition, the clinical status is evaluated, and appropriate management steps are undertaken. Finally, routine follow-up visits are scheduled as per disease requirements and clinical management guidelines.

Virtual Clinics in IR

Given the context of the pandemic over the last 3 years and the ever-evolving need to convert as much of patient care virtually as is feasible and possible, many clinics have made flexible their practice and have begun to see increasing patients via video or telephone assessment. In particular, initial assessments and visits centered around going over the results of diagnostic and therapeutic interventions, and studies can be well adapted to an online format, and so many clinics are now completing a bulk of follow-up visits without the need for the patient to physically be in office. In addition, there is an increasing amount of patients that are becoming more comfortable with this idea given the almost identical care delivered in both clinical and virtual settings. This does not, however, translate well for all patients, and there are still situations where an assessment needs to be completed in person, particularly in very ill and complex individuals where a more thorough physical assessment is necessary. In these patients the benefits, including infection prevention and control and convenience, do not justify virtual follow-up.

Summary

IR clinics are an important component of the current standard of care in IR, and an increasing number of institutions are currently implementing or have already established this practice. Further implementation and widespread adoption of outpatient IR clinics is essential for effective management of patients improving continuity in patient care experience and maintaining a strong and valued presence of IR in the field of medicine.

Acknowledgment We would like to thank Dr. Lazar Milovanovic for his contributions to this chapter (information given on first page of chapter).

References

1. Siskin GP, Bagla S, Sansivero GE, Mitchell NL. The interventional radiology clinic: key ingredients for success. J Vasc Interv Radiol. 2004;15(7):681–8.
2. Practice guideline for interventional clinical practice. Collaborative statement from the American College of Radiology, the American Society of Interventional and Therapeutic Neuroradiology, and the Society of Interventional Radiology. J Vasc Interv Radiol. 2005;16(2):149–5.
3. Murphy TP. American college of radiology practice guidelines for interventional clinical practice: a commitment to patient care. J Vasc Interv Radiol. 2005;16:157–9.
4. Katzen BT. Interventional radiology: transformation into a clinical discipline. J Am Coll Radiol. 2005;2(9):725–31.

5. Baerlocher MO, Asch MR. The future interventional radiologist: clinician or hired gun? J Vasc Interv Radiol. 2004;15(12):1385–90.
6. Murphy TP. Clinical interventional radiology: serving the patient. J Vasc Interv Radiol. 2003;14:401–3.
7. Cazzato RL, de Rubeis G, de Marini P, et al. Interventional radiology outpatient clinics (IROC): clinical impact and patient satisfaction. Cardiovasc Intervent Radiol. 2020;44(1):118–26.
8. Siskin G. Outpatient care of the interventional radiology patient. Semin Interv Radiol. 2006;23(4):337–45.

Part II
Techniques

Chapter 7
Biopsy and Drainage

Lazar Milovanovic and Ashis Bagchee-Clark

Percutaneous Needle Biopsy

PNB involves the placement of a needle into a suspected pathologic lesion in order to collect tissue or cellular samples for diagnostic clarification. There are two types of PNB, FNA and CNB, which have different indications and collect different types of tissue samples.

FNA involves inserting a very small hollow needle into the target lesion to acquire cells for cytologic evaluation [1]. CNB involves inserting a slightly larger hollow needle into the target lesion to acquire tissue for histologic evaluation [1]. In general, FNA is completed using 22 gauge needles or smaller, while CNB is completed using 20 gauge needles or larger [1]. Both CNB and FNA are completed under image guidance, which can be done using ionizing radiation (computed tomography, fluoroscopy) or non-ionizing radiation (magnetic resonance imaging, ultrasound).

A third type, vacuum-assisted core biopsy (VAB), can be described as CNB with vacuum assistance in sample collection, which results in a greater yield of tissue volume, decreasing sampling error, but also renders VAB the more invasive of the two [2]. Along with CNB, VAB sees significant use acquiring tissue from breast lesions, since excision biopsies have been replaced with percutaneous techniques as the standard of treatment [2].

Regardless of type, a percutaneous biopsy is considered successful if the collected material is adequate in order for pathologic diagnosis and treatment decisions to be made [1]. Major factors determining the likelihood of success of PNB are adequate pre-procedural and post-procedural management as well as proper patient selection based on indications.

L. Milovanovic · A. Bagchee-Clark (✉)
Michael G. DeGroote School of Medicine, McMaster University, Hamilton, ON, Canada
e-mail: lazar.milovanovic@medportal.ca; ashis.bagcheeclark@medportal.ca

S. Athreya, M. Albahhar (eds.), *Demystifying Interventional Radiology*,
https://doi.org/10.1007/978-3-031-12023-7_7

Indications for PNB

Along with excisional and open biopsy, percutaneous needle biopsy is one approach for collecting samples for pathologic characterization of lesions. Determining the most effective way to collect samples in a particular patient is done in conjunction with the most responsible physician and the radiologist.

Common indications for PNB include:

- Determination of whether a suspected tumor is benign or malignant; in the case of the latter, classification of the malignancy and staging of the patient [3]
- Collection of organic material for microbiological or genetic analysis in individuals with known or suspected infection or suspected neoplastic lesions [3]
- Identification, characterization, and spread of diffuse parenchymal diseases, such as glomerulonephritis, liver cirrhosis, or idiopathic pulmonary fibrosis (Figs. 7.1, 7.2, and 7.3) [1, 3, 4]
- Collecting material for genetic analysis [3]

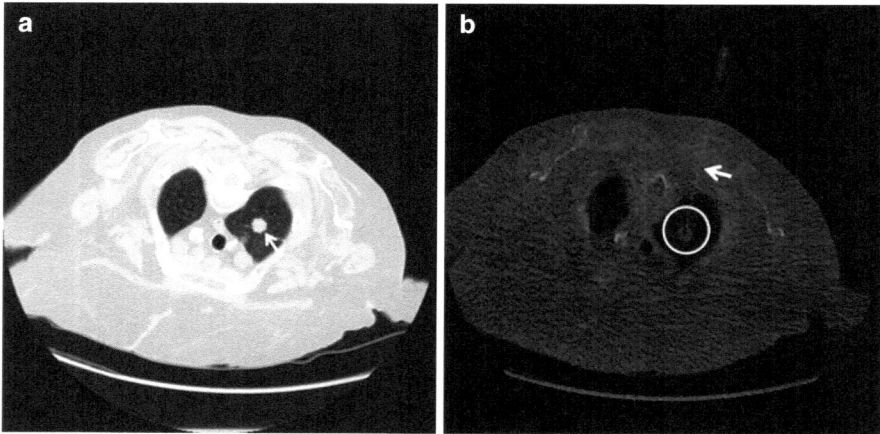

Fig. 7.1 (**a**) Soft tissue nodule (solid arrow) within the right lung apex. (**b**) CT-guided percutaneous lung biopsy of the right apical nodule (circle) with visualized biopsy needle tract (solid arrow)

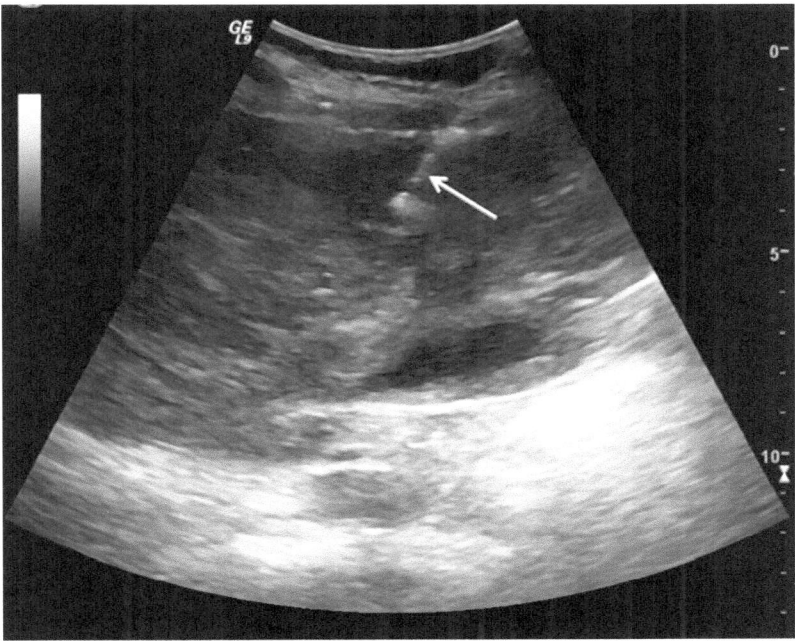

Fig. 7.2 Ultrasound-guided percutaneous needle biopsy of cirrhotic liver with visible needle tract (arrow)

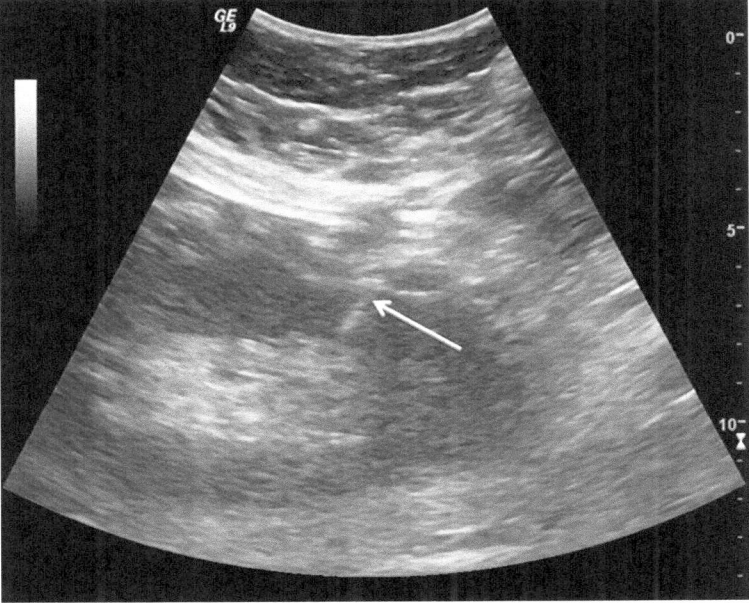

Fig. 7.3 Ultrasound-guided percutaneous needle biopsy of kidney with visible needle tract (arrow)

Contraindications for PNB

Due to the benign nature of the procedure and the decreased morbidity and mortality over alternative procedures for biopsy [1], there are few absolute contraindications for PNB; those that exist include:

- Uncorrectable significant coagulopathy [3]
- Absence of safe route for access to the lesion [3]
- Lack of consent [3]

Specific contraindications can differ based on the nature of the operation. Relative contraindications include:

- Medical conditions including coagulopathy or hemodynamic instability, including compromised cardiopulmonary function [1, 3].
- Patient parameters include uncooperative patients or inability to position the patient appropriately for the procedure [1].
- Pregnancy is a relative contraindication when ionizing radiation (CT, fluoroscopy) is used for image guidance.

Procedure

The following is a step-by-step outline of the procedure for PNB:

- A targeting scan is completed and evaluated to determine procedural approach and image guidance to be used.
- CT, MR, or ultrasound modalities can all be used for image guidance during these procedures.
- The patient is placed in the appropriate position based on the location to be biopsied and is then prepped and draped under sterile conditions.
- A local anesthetic is applied to the planned access point and expected needle path [1].
- In addition to local anesthetic, moderate sedation is occasionally used (see Chap. 5 for discussion of sedation medications).
- Under image guidance using CT or ultrasound, the guide needle is placed into the target region (Figs. 7.2 and 7.3).

- The biopsy gun with a biopsy needle is placed through the guide needle into the target region where multiple biopsy samples are then taken.
- Occasionally the guide needle is repositioned to sample multiple areas within the region of interest.
- Following removal of the guide needle, the patient is scanned post-procedure for immediate complications including bleeding and pneumothorax in lung biopsy [1].

Outcomes

Technical success of PNB is defined as the acquisition of sufficient tissue or cell material for conclusive diagnosis [1]. Expected rates of clinical and technical success for PNB of specific organs are based on Society of Interventional Radiology (SIR) Guidelines and are summarized in Table 7.1 [1].

Procedural factors affecting the success rate of PNB include number of samples collected, the experience and availability of pathology staff, type of imaging guidance used, and operator experience. Patient and lesion factors affecting the success rate of PNB include the size of the lesion to be biopsied, the organ system in which the lesion is located, and whether the lesion is benign or malignant [1].

Table 7.1 Reported and threshold success rates for specific organ systems based on SIR percutaneous needle biopsy guidelines

Biopsy site	Reported success rate (%)	Suggested threshold rate (%)
Thorax/lung	77–96	75
Musculoskeletal	76–93	70
Other sites (mediastinum, adrenal gland, head, and neck)	70–90	75

Adapted from [1]

Complications

The complications of PNB depend on the body region and organ system biopsied as well as the method of biopsy including the needle type and the use of ionizing radiation. The quantity of ionizing radiation to which the patient is exposed under CT and fluoroscopic guidance is very low, and radiation-related complications are very rare. In particular, low-dose radiation protocols are currently being introduced and are further reducing patient radiation dose [5].

Complications of IR procedures can be categorized using the Society of Interventional Radiology's two-part classification system. Part A involves a descriptive narrative of the adverse event and determination of the severity of the event itself. A "1" is considered a mild adverse event, where either no or nominal therapy is needed; a "2" is considered a moderate adverse event and involves escalation of care up to intervention under conscious sedations, blood products, and overnight admission; a "3" involves hospital admission >24 h, atypical hospital admission for the procedure, or inpatient transfer to a floor that allows for a greater level of care; a "4" indicates a disabling or life-threatening event, such as cardiopulmonary arrest; and a "5" is considered a patient death or unexpected abortion [6]. Part B allows analysis of the adverse event for quality improvement in IR and is summarized in Table 7.2 [6].

A summary of the reported complication rates and suggested threshold complications for non-thoracic and thoracic biopsies based on the 2010 SIR Guidelines is presented in Tables 7.3 and 7.4, respectively [1].

Table 7.2 Part B of the Society of Interventional Radiology's 2017 classification system of adverse events

Element of AE analysis	Category 1	Category 2	Category 3
A. Causality	AE not caused by the procedure	Unknown whether AE was caused by the procedure	AE caused by the procedure
B. Patient and procedural risk modifier	High-risk patient and technically challenging procedure	High-risk patient or low-risk patient and technically challenging procedure	No modifier
C. AE preventability	Rarely preventable	Potentially preventable	Consistently preventable
D. AE management	Most operators would have handled the AE similarly	Some operators would have handled the AE differently	Most operators would have handled the AE differently

Adapted from [6]

Table 7.3 Major complication rates for non-thoracic PNB with threshold recommendations

Major complication	Complication rate (%)	Threshold rate (%)
Bleeding[a]		
Kidney (>18 gauge)	2.7–6.6	10
Kidney (≤18 gauge)	0.5–2.8	5
Liver	0.3–3.3	5
Spleen	0–8.3	10
Others (adrenal, abdo)	0.1–3	6
Biopsy tract seeding	0–3.4	5
Pneumothorax requiring intervention	0.5	1

Adapted from [1]
[a] Transfusion or intervention is required abdo abdomen

Table 7.4 Complication rates for thoracic PNB with threshold recommendations

Complication	Severity	Complication rate (%)	Threshold rate (%)
Hemoptysis requiring hospitalization or therapy	Major	0.5	2
Thoracostomy tube placement leading to extended admission, catheter exchange, or intervention (pleurodesis)	Major	1–2	3
Air embolism	Major	0.06–0.07	<0.1
Pneumothorax	Minor	12–45	45
Thoracostomy tube placement	Minor	2–15	20

Adapted from [1]

Drainage and Aspiration

Image-guided percutaneous drainage and aspiration have become standard approaches for both therapeutic and diagnostic purposes [7]. Drainage and aspiration can be image-guided using ionizing radiation (CT, fluoroscopy) or nonionizing radiation (MRI, US). Selection of imaging modality depends on the patient, anatomical location of fluid collection, and technical difficulty of the procedure [7, 8].

Drainage involves the insertion and positioning of one or more temporary or permanent catheters via transcutaneous or trans-orifice route for ongoing drainage of fluid from a fluid collection or abscess primarily for therapeutic purposes [7]. Common transorificial routes are peroral (through the mouth), transrectal, and transvaginal [9].

Image-guided percutaneous aspiration is the extraction of part or all of the fluid within a fluid collection using a needle or a catheter [7]. In contrast to image-guided percutaneous drainage, which is primarily therapeutic, aspiration is often done with diagnostic intent and always involves removal of the needle or catheter immediately concluding the procedure [7].

Identifying Abnormal Fluid Collections and Abscesses

The decision to drain fluid collections is based on the need for diagnostic characterization and clinical assessment of symptoms [10]. Objective diagnostic imaging findings can be used to characterize fluid collections and may serve in conjunction with clinical assessment to plan intervention and future treatment. The differential for fluid collections is broad and can include abscess, hematoma, lymphocele, biloma (intra-abdominal), and seroma (postoperative) [10].

Characteristics of infected and uninfected intra-abdominal fluid collections are listed in Table 7.5 [10].

Table 7.5 Characteristics of infected and uninfected intra-abdominal fluid collections [10]

Characteristic	Adjusted odds ratio for infection
Presence of gas	32.0
Average CT density 20 HU or larger	10.0
Fluid collection wall thickness	Not associated with infection
Fluid heterogeneity and composition	Not associated with infection

HU Hounsfield unit

Indications for Drainage and/or Aspiration

The indications for drainage and aspiration as developed in the SIR standards of practice [9] are very general due to the breadth of pathology that may present as fluid collections and abscesses. An abnormal fluid collection must be present for there to be an indication to perform a procedure. Indications include:

- A general requirement for characterizing the fluid or a clinical suspicion the fluid is infected [9].
- Clinical suspicion the fluid collection is resulting from an abnormal fistula [9].
- Signs and symptoms of infection including fever, chills, leukocytosis, pain in the area of the abscess, or other severe symptoms potentially due to fluid collection [9].
- Stabilization pre-procedure or to improve subsequent procedure or intervention outcome [9].

Contraindications for Drainage and/or Aspiration

As with percutaneous needle biopsy, there are no defined absolute contraindications to percutaneous drainage and aspiration. The decision to proceed with percutaneous or surgical drainage and aspiration is made based on patient, pathology, and technical factors by the team of clinicians responsible for care of the patient [7]. Relative contraindications include:

- Medical conditions including significant uncorrectable coagulopathy or hemodynamic instability, including compromised cardiopulmonary function [7].
- Procedural parameters include absence of a safe access pathway for the lesion [7].
- Patient parameters include uncooperative patients or inability to position the patient appropriately for the procedure [7].
- Pregnancy is a relative contraindication when ionizing radiation (CT, fluoroscopy) is used for image guidance.
- General anesthesia may be required in place of moderate sedation most frequently used by diagnostic radiologists due to patient factors including allergies to anesthetic agents, cardiopulmonary instability, inability to manage airway, and pain [8].

Procedure (Fig. 7.4)

An outline of the procedure for image-guided percutaneous drainage is presented below:

- Once the decision to proceed with image-guided percutaneous drainage has been made, target imaging is used to plan the procedural approach including patient position, imaging modality (CT or ultrasound), and specific equipment.
- The patient is placed in the appropriate position, prepped and draped in a sterile manner.
- A local anesthetic is applied to the planned access point and expected needle path [1].
- In addition to local anesthetic, moderate sedation is occasionally used (see Chap. 5 for discussion of sedation medications).
- Under image guidance, a sheathed needle is used to enter the fluid collection.
- The Seldinger technique is often used to place a guidewire into the fluid collection prior to large-bore needle or catheter placement for aspiration or drainage, respectively [11].

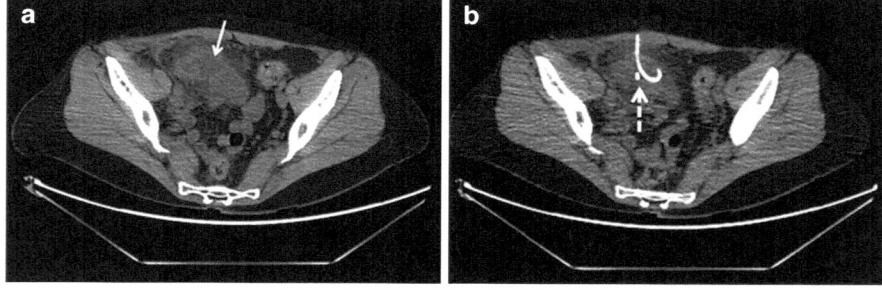

Fig. 7.4 (**a**) Thick-wall collection (solid arrow) in the right lower abdomen. (**b**) Pigtail catheter inserted under CT guidance into the abscess collection (dashed arrow)

- A portion of the fluid collection is aspirated, and often a sample may be sent for diagnostic assessment.
- One or more catheters are then placed into the fluid collection and are left to drain.
- The catheter position is evaluated on imaging, and it is sutured at the skin surface to secure the catheter in place.
- Post-procedure imaging is completed to confirm satisfactory position of the drainage catheter and assess for procedural complications.

Concerning percutaneous drainage and aspiration in pediatric populations, the techniques are relatively conserved compared to adult populations [9]. One point of note is that the body habitus of children allows for improved imaging of fluid collections, and consequently, ultrasound is more commonly able to guide drainage and aspiration procedures in pediatrics, limiting radiation exposure for the child [9].

Outcomes

The success rates of image-guided procedures of fluid collections are shown in Table 7.6, as adapted from the Society of Interventional Radiology Quality Improvement Guideline for Drainage/Aspiration of Abscesses [9]. Success rates depended on whether the aim was diagnostic aspiration or drainage [9]. With respect to therapeutic drainage, "curative" drainage was defined as infection resolution with no subsequent interventions; "partial success" was defined as drainage of the abscess with subsequent intervention necessitated [9].

Table 7.6 Success rates of image-guided percutaneous procedures of fluid collections, adapted from [9]

Outcome	Reported rate (%)
Successful diagnostic fluid aspiration: Aspiration of fluid adequate for diagnostic characterization	93–100
Successful drainage: Curative and partial success	62–100

Complications

The complications of fluid drainage and aspiration depend on the characteristics of the fluid, the location of the fluid collection (Table 7.7) [8], patient comorbidities, technical factors including procedural difficulty, and type of imaging used.

Common complications include infection (both those which were present before drainage and those caused by continued catheter placement), bleeding, and puncture of adjacent critical structures [12]. Adverse events in those undergoing image-guided percutaneous drainage and aspiration are reported in up to 15% of patients [9].

Table 7.7 Complications for drainage and aspiration by body region [7]

Body region	Fluid collection types	Common and major complications	Complication risk factors
Thorax	Empyema, lung abscess, mediastinal abscess, sterile pleural effusion	Pneumothorax, fluid loculation, septation of collection area	Bronchopleural fistula, large pleural leak, hemothorax
Abdomen	Liver abscess, spleen abscess, perforated viscus resulting in fluid accumulation	Hepatocolic fistula creation, sepsis, puncture of adjacent structures, bleeding, death by biliary peritonitis	Transpleural drainage
Pancreas, kidney, retroperitoneal space	Pancreatic collections from pancreatitis or duct injury, renal and perinephric fluid collections	Fistula formation, hemorrhage, infection, sepsis	None characterized
Pelvis	Pelvic abscess	Hemorrhage, pain, introduction of colonic or vaginal flora into sterile fluid	None characterized

References

1. Gupta S, Wallace MJ, Cardella JF, Kundu S, Miller DL, Rose SC. Quality improvement guidelines for percutaneous needle biopsy. J Vasc Interv Radiol. 2010;21:969–75.
2. Nakano S, Imawari Y, Mibu A, Otsuka M, Oinuma T. Differentiating vacuum-assisted breast biopsy from core needle biopsy: is it necessary? Br J Radiol. 2018;91(1092):20180250.
3. Veltri A, Bargellini I, Giorgi L, Almeida PA, Akhan O. CIRSE guidelines on percutaneous needle biopsy (PNB). Cardiovasc Intervent Radiol. 2017;40(10):1501–13.
4. Vijayaraghavan GR, David S, Bermudez-Allende M, Sarwat H. Imaging-guided parenchymal liver biopsy: how we do it. J Clin Imaging Sci. 2011;1:30.
5. Adiga S, Athreya S. Safety, efficacy, and feasibility of an ultra-low dose radiation protocol for CT-guided percutaneous needle biopsy of pulmonary lesions: initial experience. Clin Radiol. 2014;69(7):709–14.
6. Khalilzadeh O, Baerlocher MO, Shyn PB, Connolly BL, Devane AM, Morris CS, Cohen AM, Midia M, Thornton RH, Gross K, Caplin DM. Proposal of a new adverse event classification by the Society of Interventional Radiology Standards of Practice Committee. J Vasc Interv Radiol. 2017;28(10):1432–7.
7. Wallace MJ, Chin KW, Fletcher TB, et al. Quality improvement guidelines for percutaneous drainage/aspiration of abscess and fluid collections. J Vasc Interv Radiol. 2010;21:431–5.
8. Lorenz J, Thomas JL. Complications of percutaneous fluid drainage. Semin Interv Radiol. 2006;23(2):194–204.
9. Dariushnia SR, Mitchell JW, Chaudry G, Hogan MJ. Society of interventional radiology quality improvement standards for image-guided percutaneous drainage and aspiration of abscesses and fluid collections. J Vasc Interv Radiol. 2020;31(4):662–6.
10. Allen BC, Barnhart H, Bashir M, Nieman C, Breault S, Jaffe TA. Diagnostic accuracy of intraabdominal fluid collection characterized in the era of multidetector computed tomography. Am Surg. 2012;78(2):185–9.
11. Seldinger SI. Catheter replacement of the needle in percutaneous arteriography; a new technique. Acta Radiol. 1953;39(5):368–76.
12. Winokur RS, Pua BB, Sullivan BW, Madoff DC. Percutaneous lung biopsy: technique, efficacy and complications. Semin Interv Radiol. 2013;30(2):121–7.

Chapter 8
Arterial and Venous Access

Eva Liu and Jason Martin

Arterial Access

The purpose of arterial access is to provide adequate and safe entry to the vasculature. Several factors should be considered prior to obtaining arterial access.

General principles of vascular access [1, 2]:

1. Pre-operative planning requires the operator to choose a puncture site appropriate to patient anatomy, operator expertise, and requirements of the procedure.
2. When deciding on the site of a diagnostic procedure, take into account that endovascular intervention may be required.
3. Prior to puncture, make sure to relate the site to anatomical landmarks.
4. Use a standardized, reproducible technique.
5. If you encounter problems, do not be afraid to switch sites.

Although several puncture sites are available, for the sake of this chapter, we will focus on techniques for femoral access.

E. Liu (✉)
Michael G. DeGroote School of Medicine, McMaster University, Hamilton, ON, Canada
e-mail: eva.liu@medportal.ca

J. Martin
Department of Medical Imaging, University of Toronto, Toronto, ON, Canada
e-mail: jason.martin@medportal.ca

© The Author(s), under exclusive license to Springer Nature Switzerland AG 2022
S. Athreya, M. Albahhar (eds.), *Demystifying Interventional Radiology*,
https://doi.org/10.1007/978-3-031-12023-7_8

Anatomy

Identifying the proper puncture site is key to obtaining proper arterial access as most complications occur at the puncture site itself. The femoral artery passes beneath the inguinal ligament which extends from the anterior superior iliac spine (ASIS) to the pubic tubercle [2]. Fluoroscopy may be used to locate the head of the femur as an anatomical landmark. The artery usually passes along the medial side of the femoral head [2]. Beware of using groin creases as a landmark, as in obese patients, these may be increasingly distal to the inguinal ligament [2].

Procedure

The potential location of the common femoral artery is evaluated by tracing along the inguinal ligament [2]. The femoral artery can be landmarked to be 2/3 between the ASIS and the pubic tubercle. Ultrasound can be used to guide the proper landmarking of the artery. After applying the ultrasound probe to the appropriate landmark, pressure can be applied using the ultrasound probe to distinguish the non-compressible femoral artery from the compressible femoral vein. Once the bifurcation of the femoral artery has been identified, the probe can move more proximally to identify the common femoral artery. The artery is trapped between the index and middle finger using the operator's nondominant hand [2]. Lidocaine (1%) is injected into the skin and subcutaneous tissues between the index and middle finger. Penetration of the local anesthetic causes the femoral pulse to be appreciated more clearly [2].

The artery is approached using an entry needle at a 45° angle, and the needle is advanced through the anterior wall of the artery (Figs. 8.1, 8.2, and 8.3). Once pulsatile bleeding is achieved through the needle, the nondominant hand may be used to secure the needle [2]. The floppy-tip portion of the guidewire may be advanced through the needle, and placement is confirmed using fluoroscopy [2]. A 1–2 mm

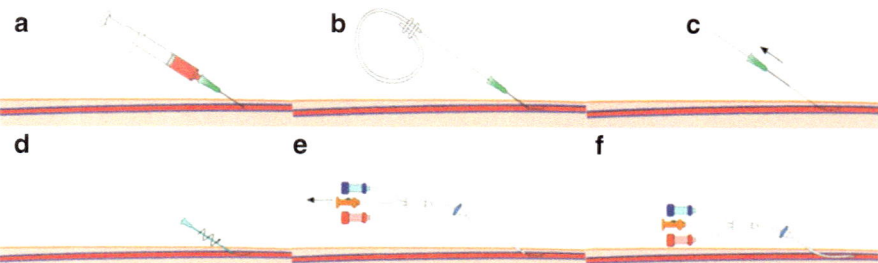

Fig. 8.1 The Seldinger technique (**a–f**)

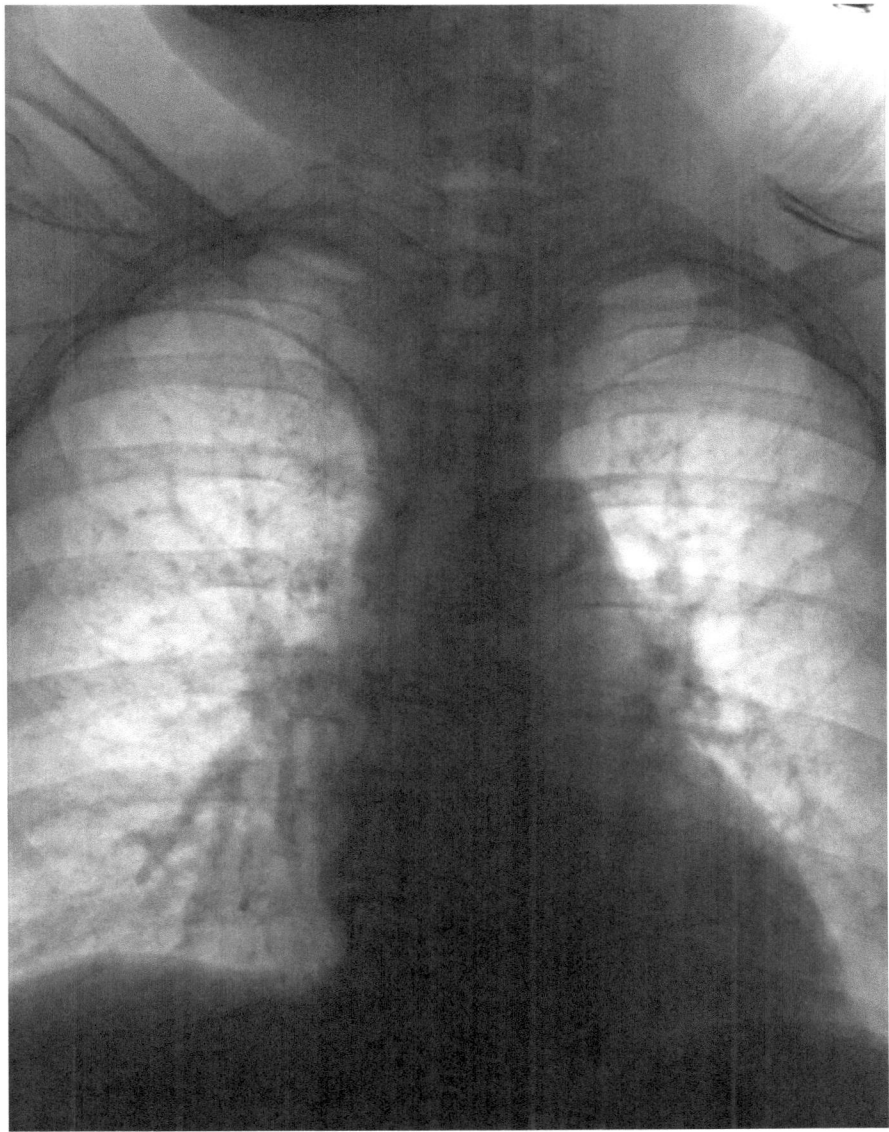

Fig. 8.2 Chest radiograph revealing tunneled dialysis catheter in place

incision is created in the area of the injection, and a mosquito clamp can be used to dilate the puncture site [2]. The needle can then be removed and exchanged for a sheath [2]. Hemostasis at the end of the procedure can either be achieved with a percutaneous closure device or firm compression of the artery for 10–15 min.

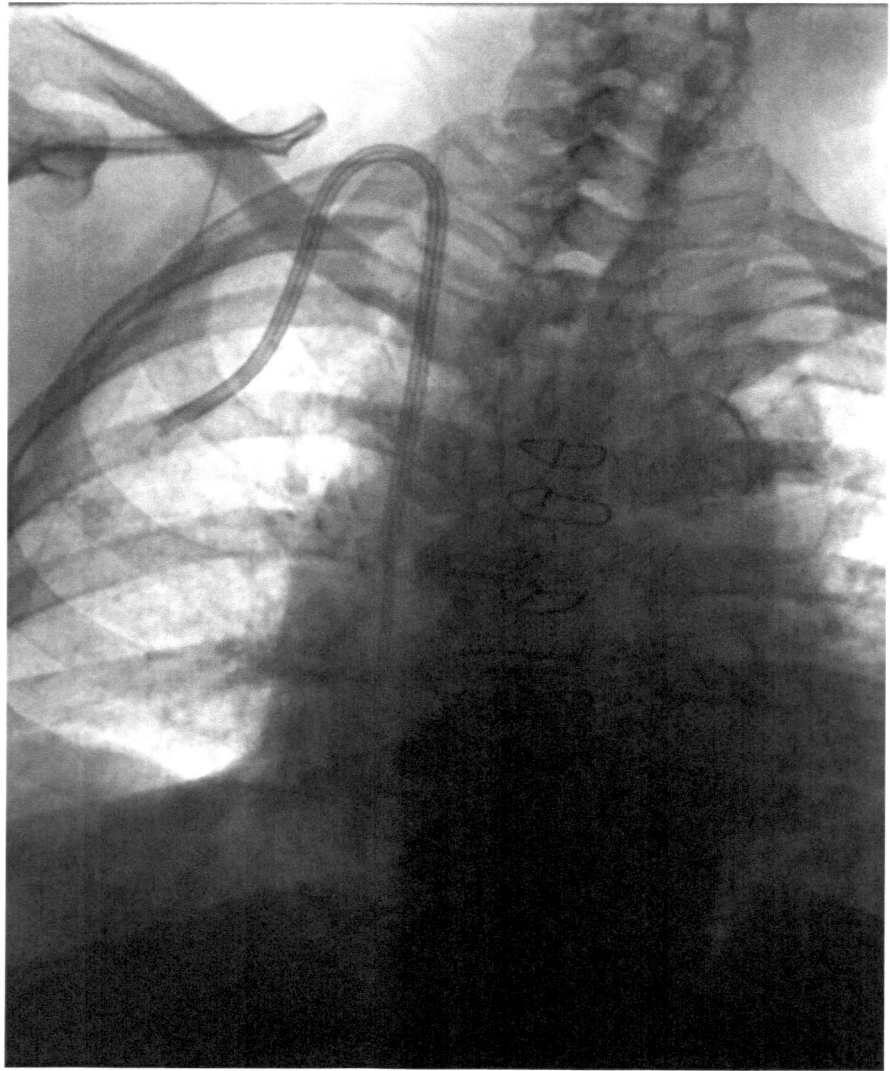

Fig. 8.3 Chest radiograph revealing PICC line in right brachial vein extending to the cavoatrial junction

Complications

Groin hematoma is a complication after femoral access that can range from minor to major. Most groin hematomas can be controlled with manual compression for 10–15 min and frequent check to make sure that the hematoma softens and does not continue to evolve in size [3].

Arteriovenous fistula is another possible complication after femoral access associated with low puncture at the level of the bifurcation. This complication is rarely symptomatic but can cause heart failure, lower extremity edema, and arterial insufficiency in rare cases. Diagnosis is made with ultrasound. Treatment ranges from observation to endovascular exclusion and surgical intervention [3].

Pseudoaneurysm is another complication of femoral access. Femoral pseudoaneurysms are results of insufficient sealing of the closure site and communication between the femoral artery and the overlying hematoma. Diagnosis can be made with ultrasound. Treatment ranges from observation, thrombin injection, and endovascular to surgical intervention [3].

Retroperitoneal bleed is the most life-threatening complication after femoral access. Patients typically present with suprainguinal fullness, severe back and lower quadrant abdominal pain, femoral neuropathy, and hypotension. Diagnosis is best made with computed tomography with contrast, and treatment includes blood transfusion and endovascular or surgical intervention [3].

Venous Access

Conventional Peripheral IV Lines

Conventional peripheral intravenous lines are cheap, effective, and used for short-term access. Complication rates of phlebitis and infection increase substantially with increased catheter dwell time; therefore, replacement should occur every 3–4 days [4, 5].

Central Catheters

Central Lines

There are no absolute contraindications to using central lines, as they can be lifesaving. Indications include administration of IV fluid, medications or blood products, inaccessible peripheral veins, repeated blood sampling, or vein-irritating medication such as chemotherapy. They are mainly placed in the internal and external jugular, although subclavian access may be used [4, 5].

There are three types of centrally inserted catheters:

1. Non-tunneled

    • Used for short-term access for rapid resuscitation or pressure monitoring.
    • Life span is 5–7 days.
    • Higher infection risk.

2. Skin-tunneled

   • Good for longer dwell times
   • Used in patients requiring long-term dialysis and frequent IV access, especially for blood products

3. Implantable ports

   • Catheter attached to reservoir implanted into surgically created pocket in the chest wall. A needle may be placed into the reservoir to attain access.
   • Less interference with daily activity, less flushing, reduced risk of infection.
   • Expensive to insert and difficult to remove.

Peripherally Inserted Central Catheters (PICCs)

PICCs are indicated for use in patients requiring several weeks to 6 months of IV therapy. This usually includes peripheral delivery of nutrition, antibiotics, analgesics, chemotherapy, or blood products. They are inserted into the basilic, cephalic, or brachial veins and rest in the cavoatrial junction. Insertion of PICCs is safer than central lines, with minimal risk of pneumothorax and hemothorax. Complications include loss of placement, occlusion, deep vein thrombosis (DVT), or phlebitis [4, 5].

Infections

Differentiating between local site inflammation and true infection is crucial. Infections can include site cellulitis, skin tract or tunnel infection, and bacteremia. Prophylactic antibiotics have not been shown to decrease infection rates [4, 5].

Acknowledgment We would like to thank Dr. Jason Martin for his contributions to this chapter (information given on first page of chapter).

References

1. Kessel D, Robertson I. Interventional radiology: a survival guide. 2nd ed. Philadelphia: Elsevier; 2005.
2. Schneider PA. Endovascular skills—guidewire and catheter skills for endovascular surgery. 2nd ed. New York: Marcel Dekker; 2003.
3. Stone PA, Campbell JE. Complications related to femoral artery access for transcatheter procedures. Vasc Endovasc Surg. 2012;46(8):617–23.
4. Cheung E, Baerlocher MO, Asch M, Myers A. Venous access: a practical review for 2009. Can Fam Physician. 2009;55(5):494–6.
5. Dougherty L. Central venous access devices. Oxford: Blackwell; 2006.

Chapter 9
Embolization Materials and Principles

Eva Liu, Ashis Bagchee-Clark, and Jason Martin

Indications

The constellation of medical conditions treated with embolization continues to grow. Control of hemorrhage is a common indication for embolization [1]. The range of hemorrhagic indications for embolization include gastrointestinal tract bleeds, retroperitoneal bleeds, hemoptysis, postpartum hemorrhage, hemorrhage post surgery, and traumatic hemorrhage, such as pelvic fracture [1].

Another common use for embolization is in occluding an artery to reduce or stop blood supply to a specific area and, as a consequence of this, shrink or prevent further development of a growth in that area [1]. Examples of this include embolization to treat renal cell carcinoma, hepatocellular carcinoma, arteriovenous malformations, and uterine fibroids [1]. Newer indications include prostate artery embolization (PAE) for benign prostatic enlargement (BPH), genicular artery embolization for osteoarthritis, and hemorrhoidal artery embolization for hemorrhoids. In an analogous fashion, embolization also sees utility in diverting blood away from a specific pathology. An example of this is varicocele embolization, where blood is routed away from enlarged scrotal veins, thus relieving pain, swelling, and potential infertility [1].

Aneurysms can also be treated through embolization, with the option to either divert blood from the weakened artery or induce clotting within the aneurysmal segment [1]. This demonstrates the broad utility of embolization.

E. Liu (✉) · A. Bagchee-Clark
Michael G. DeGroote School of Medicine, McMaster University, Hamilton, ON, Canada
e-mail: eva.liu@medportal.ca; ashis.bagcheeclark@medportal.ca

J. Martin
Department of Medical Imaging, University of Toronto, Toronto, ON, Canada
e-mail: jason.martin@medportal.ca

Embolization Agents (Liquids, Particles, Gelfoam, and Coils)

Embolization agents can be categorized into temporary and permanent agents. Temporary agents include Gelfoam. Permanent agents include coils and particles. Most liquid agents have no role in traumatic embolization due to increased risk of tissue necrosis [2, 3].

Particles

Particles, or particulates, were the first embolic agents developed and are still the most commonly used owing in large part to their versatility; particulates can have a calibrated shape, provide a temporary or permanent embolism, and can be natural or synthetic by design [4].

Particles adhere to the vessel wall and cause mechanical occlusion and an inflammatory reaction. Common particles include polyvinyl alcohol (PVA), trisacryl gelatin microspheres (TAGM), and hydrogel. Sizes range by 200 μm: 100–300 μm, 300–500 μm, 500–700 μm, 700–900 μm, and 900–1200 μm [2, 3].

Particles are mixed with saline and contrast, and a three-way stopcock is used to mix the solution. Frequent remixing is important to prevent particle aggregation, which increases as more contrast is used [2, 3].

Polyvinyl Alcohol (PVA) Particulates

PVA particulates are a biocompatible polymer and are permanently occlusive as a consequence [4]. Common indications for embolization using PVA particulates include arteriovenous malformations, lower gastrointestinal bleeding, and bone metastases [4].

Ranging from 100 to 1100 μm, the varying sizes of PVA particles give rise to a disadvantage where particles potentially aggregate in a more proximal fashion than planned [4].

Calibrated Microspheres

Microspheres of calibrated and thus more consistent size help reduce one of the major drawbacks of PVA particles, namely, the unwanted embolization of proximal blood vessels [4]. The calibrated nature also allows the production of microspheres of various sizes which enables more targeted and distal embolizations [4].

Gelatin Sponge Particles

Gelatin sponge is a temporary embolization agent made of purified skin gelatin. It is used commonly in trauma or to provide distal embolization with subsequent proximal embolization with coils. Gastrointestinal bleeding and uterine fibroids are also commonly treated with gelatin sponges [4].

It is inexpensive and readily available and is a temporary vessel recanalization after gelfoam embolization is seen within 2 weeks, but can take up to 4 months for maximum restoration [1, 5]. Unintentional permanent occlusion can potentially occur due to intimal thickening as a consequence of an inflammatory response [4].

Disadvantages include nonuniform particle size, and clot disruption with rebleeding is possible.

Liquid Agents

Liquid agents are favorable in embolization as they do not rely on the patient's own coagulation system and therefore can be used in patients with severe coagulopathy. They can also be used to embolize sites distal to the catheter which is useful when the target cannot be reached with the catheter. The disadvantage is that liquid embolization agents are difficult to control and require higher operator expertise [6].

Liquid agents include absolute alcohol (ethanol), N-butyl cyanoacrylate (NBCA), and ethylene vinyl alcohol copolymer (Onyx) [7]. Ethanol is a commonly used sclerosing agent that causes protein denaturation and permanent vascular occlusion [7]. Indication for ethanol embolization includes renal tumor ablation and portal vein embolization. NBCA and Onyx are quite expensive and work by polymerizing upon coming in contact with blood. They can be used to treat peripheral vascular malformations and pseudoaneurysms [2, 3, 6].

Thrombin

Thrombin is the last step of the coagulation cascade and can be used off-label for iatrogenic pseudoaneurysm after catheterization not amenable to conventional embolization [7]. Derived from bovine thrombin, there is a rare risk of allergic reactions. The mechanism of action includes the direct activation of fibrinogen, converting it into fibrin monomers. Thrombin does have a potential for accidental distal embolization. It can also be used for endoleak repair after aortic aneurysm endograft [2, 3].

Coils

Coils are a common embolization agent that induce embolization through mechanical obstruction and provide a prothrombotic surface for thrombus to form. They consist of steel or platinum wire looped in different sizes and orientations (Fig. 9.1). Platinum coils are more opaque and malleable than steel, but are more expensive. Bare metal coils cause incomplete occlusion as they rely solely on mechanical obstruction. Some coils have fibers (wool, nylon, silk, etc.) to increase thrombogenicity [6].

Coils should be sized based on the target vessel. Ideally, the coil should be 20–30% larger than the target vessel. Undersized coils have a risk of migration and causing distal embolization. Oversized coils have a risk of not forming appropriate coils inside the vessel which can lead to incomplete occlusion. Although coils are flexible and effective embolization devices, they do require thrombus formation and may be hindered by severe coagulopathy [6].

The Amplatzer Vascular Plug (AVP) is a commonly used mechanical embolization device that is composed of self-expanding nitinol mesh. They are relatively expensive but can be used in high flow vessels with low risk of migration. Indications for AVPs include the splenic artery, the portal vein, pulmonary arteriovenous malformations, and the internal iliac artery [6].

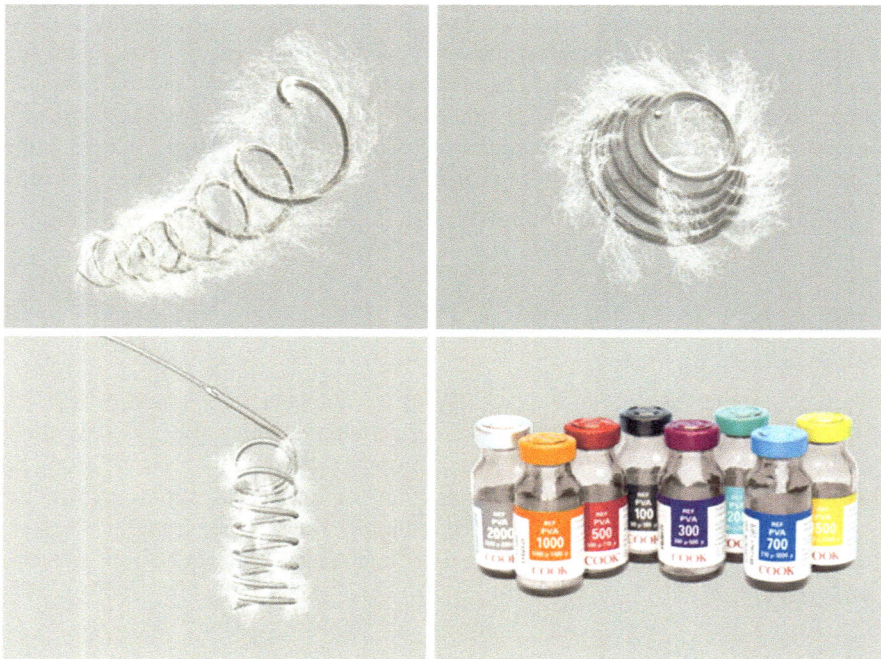

Fig. 9.1 Coils and PVA particles used in embolization

Principles: Tips and Tricks

- Always keep a separate table with the embolization material and separate bowls for saline and contrast.
- Syringes used for embolization should not be used for postembolization angiograms.
- Test contrast injections of the selected vessel should be performed to assess catheter position and the flow within the vessel for reflux potential.
- As the agent is injected, do so in small aliquots or "puffs."
- Your postembolization DSA should use the same rate and puffs to assess vascular stasis.
- After injecting the agent, flush your catheter with saline to purge the device of agent. This also prevents aggregation at the tip of the microcatheter.
- Be wary of flow as you embolize. Initially fast-flowing vessels may slow, increasing the risk of reflux.
- The lumen of your catheter contains a good amount of fluid, so as the vessel approaches stasis, understand that excessive flushing or administration of agent may cause reflux and accidental embolization of other organs.

Acknowledgment   We would like to thank Dr. Jason Martin for his contributions to this chapter (information given on first page of chapter).

References

1. Arnold MJ, Keung JJ, McCarragher B. Interventional radiology: indications and best practices. Am Fam Physician. 2019;99(9):547–56.
2. Abada HT, Golzarian J. Gelatine sponge particles: handling characteristics for endovascular use. Tech Vasc Interv Radiol. 2007;10:257–60.
3. Laurent A. Microspheres and nonspherical particles for embolization. Tech Vasc Interv Radiol. 2007;10:248–56.
4. Lopera J. Embolization in trauma: principles and techniques. Semin Interv Radiol. 2010;27:014–28.
5. Hilal SK, Michelsen JW. Therapeutic percutaneous embolization for extra-axial vascular lesions of the head, neck, and spine. J Neurosurg. 1975;43(3):275–87.
6. Medsinge A, Zajko A, Orons P, Amesur N, Santos E. A case-based approach to common embolization agents used in vascular interventional radiology. Am J Roentgenol. 2014;203(4):699–708.
7. Maybody M, Madoff DC, Thornton RH, Morales SA, Moskowitz CS, Hsu M, Brody LA, Brown KT, Covey AM. Catheter-directed endovascular application of thrombin: report of 3 cases and review of the literature. Clin Imaging. 2017;42:96–105.

Chapter 10
Image-Guided Tumor Ablative Therapies

Ashis Bagchee-Clark, Anna Hwang, and Lazar Milovanovic

Non-thermal Ablative Therapy

Chemical Ablation

Chemical ablation is a type of non-thermal ablative therapy using intratumoral injection of chemical substances including ethanol and acetic acid. These chemical substances can have both direct and indirect anti-tumor effects. As an example, percutaneous ethanol injections (PEI) can directly cause cell death through protein denaturation and cellular dehydration and, once ethanol has entered the nearby circulation, can indirectly cause tissue necrosis through tumor vasculature thrombosis [1].

Chemical ablation is an inexpensive and simple procedure that has been used in small lesions primarily in the liver [2]. It is an effective treatment modality for local tumor management in developing regions due to its low cost, few infrastructural requirements, and procedure simplicity. Success of this procedure is lower than other ablation therapies due to difficulty establishing uniform diffusion of ablative materials over the entire tumor volume. RFA has been found superior to PEI in terms of local control of small hepatocellular carcinomas and 3-year survival [3]. Currently, it is primarily utilized as an adjuvant therapy in addition to primary therapy in lesions that are difficult to treat with thermal ablation [4–6].

A. Bagchee-Clark · A. Hwang (✉) · L. Milovanovic
Michael G. DeGroote School of Medicine, McMaster University, Hamilton, ON, Canada
e-mail: ashis.bagcheeclark@medportal.ca; anna.hwang@medportal.ca;
lazar.milovanovic@medportal.ca

S. Athreya, M. Albahhar (eds.), *Demystifying Interventional Radiology*,
https://doi.org/10.1007/978-3-031-12023-7_10

Indications

- Adjuvant therapy in tumors that cannot be treated using thermal ablation techniques due to lesion size, position, or patient factors
- Small subcutaneous tumors including thyroid cancer [7]
- Management of focal benign lesions [8]
- Hepatocellular carcinoma (HCC) in patients with cirrhosis [5]

Contraindications

- Patients with uncorrectable coagulopathy
- More than three tumors in the organ to be treated
- Liver failure based on the presence of ascites and/or jaundice (for treatment of HCC)
- Metastatic lesions in the liver
- Tumor invasion of the vasculature

Procedure

- Chemical ablation is done under ultrasound or computed tomography (CT) guidance.
- The patient is placed under conscious sedation.
- The planned puncture area and expected needle path are treated with local anesthetic.
- An 18G or 19G needle is introduced into the lesion, and the tip is placed near the peripheral margin of the tumor.
- Ethanol or acetic acid is injected slowly under image guidance until treatment fluid has diffused through the tumor.
- If ethanol is used, dose is volume-dependent, but usually 2–10 mL of absolute 99.5% ethanol is used per session [5].
- If acetic acid is used, dose is volume-dependent, but usually 1–3 mL of 50% acetic acid is injected [5].

Complications

Complications can include pain, fever, a feeling of alcohol intoxication, and elevated transaminase (if using ethanol). There is also an increased risk of inappropriate vein thrombosis, for example, jugular vein thrombosis occurring after treatment of thyroid nodules with PEI [9].

Outcomes

The goal of chemical ablation is local tumor control. One-, two-, and three-year local recurrence rates were reported to be 16%, 34%, and 34% for percutaneous ethanol injection and 14%, 31%, and 31% for percutaneous acetic acid injection for HCC in a randomized control trial [5].

Irreversible Electroporation

Irreversible electroporation (IRE) is a non-thermal ablative therapy that can serve as an alternative to thermal ablative therapy in patients unable to undergo surgical resection of a tumor, often due to proximity to critical vasculature [10]. IRE functions by using a high-voltage pulsed electrical current to create an electric field which disrupts the electric potential gradient across tumor cell membranes. Disruption of the electric potential gradient leads to the creation of permanent nano-pores in the cell membrane, altering membrane permeability and cell homeostasis and leading to apoptosis. Multiple factors affect the efficacy of IRE including tissue physical parameters and electric field characteristics.

The mechanism of IRE confers it a tissue selectivity that allows it to better preserve nearby structures in the ablated region when compared to other less discriminative ablation therapies [10]. IRE is able to preserve vital structures within the ablated region due to reduced effects from IRE on the collagenous structures and pericellular matrix proteins that comprise the hepatic vasculature, portal vein, and intrahepatic bile ducts [2, 6, 11–13]. In addition to this tissue selectivity, IRE is also advantageous due to possessing sharp demarcations between ablated and non-ablated regions that are only one to two cells thick [14], short treatment times, and a lack of a heat-sink effect [10].

Indications

As IRE remains a newer less-established therapy, the indications for IRE are largely still being determined. Studies and clinical trials have examined the use of IRE in the treatment of the brain, lung, liver, kidney, pancreas, and prostate [10].

Across those clinical trials, significant therapeutic promise has been shown in using IRE to treat tumors in the prostate, pancreas, and liver, all difficult cancers to treat effectively, due in part to their apposition to other important structures [10]. For prostate cancer, IRE has demonstrated similar 5-year recurrence rates to radical prostatectomy, with greater urogenital and erectile function often observed post-treatment with IRE given the relative sparing of both the neurovascular bundle and genitourinary structures [10]. Similarly, while more studies are required to fully understand IRE's efficacy in treating pancreatic cancer, a potential role exists for IRE and its greater tissue selectivity, as the proximity of the pancreas to major vessels such as the celiac trunk and hepatic artery have resulted in significant morbidity when treated with thermal ablation [10]. Treating cancers of the liver, also in close proximity to many key vessels and vital structures, also benefits from the greater tissue selectivity seen with IRE [10]. Hepatic lesion IRE is indicated in patients with no systemic metastases and all hepatic lesions smaller than 3–4 cm [11].

Device

The most commonly used device for IRE is the AngioDynamics NanoKnife system (AngioDynamics, Latham, NY). The NanoKnife system is comprised of a computer-controlled pulse generator, a footswitch, and disposable single-use electrodes. The generator can operate with up to six probe outputs creating a maximum current of 50 A. Electric pulses are usually 3 kV in magnitude and last 20–100 ms. Variable parameters include pulse duration, electrode configuration and placement, and geometry. Spacing, position, and number of electrodes required to treat a particular tumor are calculated by the generator based on a computer algorithm.

Procedure

- Pre-treatment planning is completed based on preoperative CT scan imaging to quantify tumor volume, dimensions, and morphology.
- IRE probes are positioned in the region of interest based on calculated positions and bracket the tumor.
- This procedure is often done under general anesthesia in order to minimize motion during the procedure.
- Pulse delivery is synchronized to the absolute myocardial refractory period on the patient's ECG after the R-wave.

Outcome and Post-procedure Follow-Up

Treatment technical success is defined as successful delivery of all planned pulses based on the algorithm design after assessment of lesion dimensions and characteristics. Technical success also includes complete ablation without evidence of enhancement on axial CT scan 8 weeks post-procedure. Studies have proposed an initial follow-up of 12 weeks post-IRE therapy, then every 3-month following. Periprocedural mortality was reported at 0.6% in one multi-institutional study [11].

Complications

Complications can include [6]:

- Muscle contraction or cardiac arrhythmias secondary to electrical harmonics generated by current IRE devices
- Increased bleeding risk due to lack of coagulation around needle puncture site and tract
- Tumor recurrence due to areas of reversible electroporation within the treated area
- Deep vein thrombosis with or without pulmonary embolism
- Bile leak or biliary stricture
- Massive bleeding requiring transfusion
- Periprocedural nausea and vomiting
- Periprocedural infection
- Severe pain

Emerging Non-thermal Ablative Techniques

Histotripsy

Analogous to the thermal ablative technique of high-intensity focused ultrasound, histotripsy utilizes focused acoustic energy to create cavitation bubbles within the body and thus homogenize a targeted region of tissue into acellular debris [14]. This technique of targeted homogenization can be applied to cancerous tissue, and in the past couple of years, human trials have begun regarding histotripsy in the treatment of liver cancer.

At the moment, histotripsy is a noninvasive procedure, and thus it can be argued that it doesn't fall directly under the umbrella of interventional radiology. That said, histotripsy does utilize ultrasound, an imaging modality, to guide and monitor tissue ablation in a form that can be described as tissue erosion surgery [15]. Additionally, as catheters possessing ultrasonic transducers do exist, the idea of histotripsy eventually evolving into an image-guided minimally invasive procedure allowing more finite ablations in the body is, at the very least, possible.

Mechanochemical Ablation

Mechanochemical ablation simply combines two ablative techniques: HIFU and chemical ablation [16]. Mechanochemical ablation is a technique currently used in treating conditions such as chronic venous reflux, though, in that case, a rotating catheter is responsible for the mechanical damage and a liquid sclerosant is the chemical infusion [17].

In the treatment of cancer, mechanochemical ablation is an incredibly novel technique with little to no apparent study of the technique in humans yet. Studies using xenograft models of both prostate cancer and liver cancer have indicated that mechanochemical ablation demonstrates curative potential of said cancers [16, 18].

Thermal Ablative Therapy

Thermal ablative therapy uses heating or cooling to induce necrosis. Heating techniques include radiofrequency ablation, microwave ablation, and high-frequency ultrasound. Cooling techniques include cryoablation.

Thermal ablation is indicated in the treatment of various tumors or metastases under 5 cm that cannot be surgically resected. Choice of a modality depends on many factors including tumor size, location, and proximity to vasculature. Radiofrequency ablation (RFA) is effective for smaller tumors (<3 cm) but is limited by tissue impedance and proximity to vasculature. Microwave ablation (MWA) can cover a broader range, and its efficacy is less affected by impedance and proximity to vasculature; however it has a higher risk of complications. Cryoablation is easily visualized on imaging, allowing for better monitoring and a clearly defined treatment margin. High-intensity focused ultrasound (HIFU) is a newer modality that provides precise, noninvasive ablation to more superficial regions such as the prostate or uterus.

Radiofrequency Ablation

Radiofrequency ablation (RFA) is a well-established thermal ablation technique that utilizes frictional energy to heat the tumor tissue and cause protein denaturation leading to coagulation necrosis. Frictional energy is created from vibration of polar molecules moving in-phase with an alternating current created by radiofrequency waves created by RF electrodes placed in the tissue. In addition to heat from frictional energy, resistive heat of the tumor tissue is generated by electric current travelling through ionic tissue. RFA has been demonstrated in hepatic, renal, and pulmonary lesions for local management in nonsurgical candidates (Fig. 10.1) [4–6, 12, 19–23].

The goal of radiofrequency ablation is local tumor control and prolonged survival. Complete ablation is characterized by a non-enhancing region in the location of the tumor and ablative margin on contrast-enhanced imaging.

RFA is indicated in patients with renal, hepatic, or pulmonary primary or metastatic lesions without systemic disease as well as palliative management of benign and malignant osseous lesions.

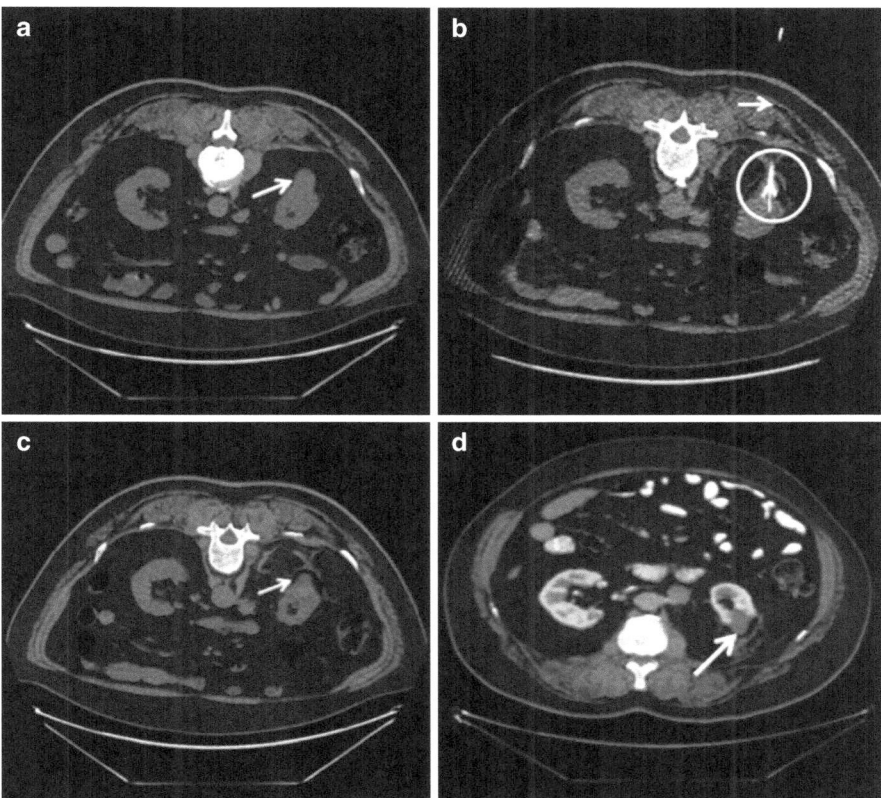

Fig. 10.1 (**a**) Exophytic renal mass (solid arrow) prior to radiofrequency ablation (RFA). (**b**) RFA probe (circle) within the right renal tumor with needle tract visible (solid arrow). (**c**) Immediate post-RFA ablation. (**d**) 12-month post-ablation zone with no tumor recurrence

Device and Technique

There are multiple different types of commercially available and currently used RFA devices: AngioDynamics (Queensbury, NY), LaVeen Boston Scientific (Natick, MA), Radionics (Burlington, MA), and Valleylab Covidien (Mansfield, MA). The RFA apparatus is comprised of an RFA generator (Fig. 10.2a), electrodes, and array (Fig. 10.2b).

There are multiple different gauge caliber electrodes available ranging from 14 to 17 gauge in caliber with variable ablation zone sizes depending on electrode parameters. The electrodes are available in different types (expandable multi-tined, internally cooled, or perfused), lengths, gauges, and tine configurations depending on the depth of tumor and patient factors.

The major difference between different types of generators is the control system: both impedance-based and temperature-based control systems are available.

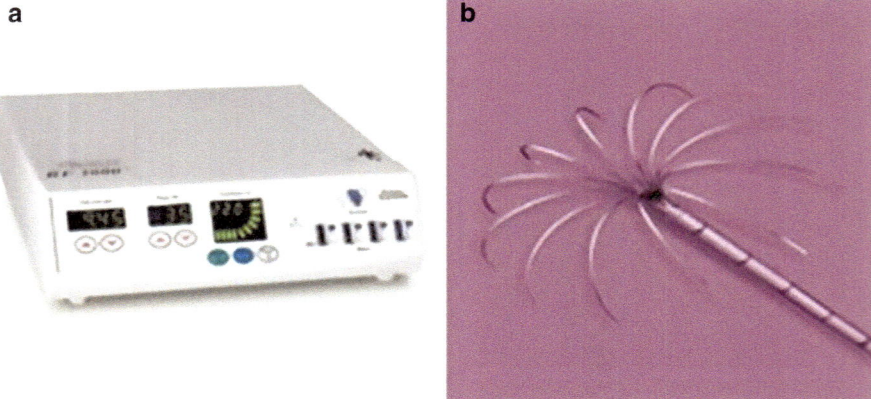

Fig. 10.2 (**a**) An impedance-driven Boston Scientific RF3000 radiofrequency generator. (**b**) A Boston Scientific RFA needle electrode with array deployed. (Figures used with permission of Boston Scientific)

Impedance-based RF generators function by applying increasing energy to the electrode until tissue desiccation occurs and the tissue impedance exceeds a pre-defined threshold [24]. Temperature-based RF generators function by delivering energy to the RF electrode in sufficient amount to increase the tissue temperature to a pre-defined level in order to cause necrosis [24]. Generally, electrodes are available from 14 to 17 gauge with single probes or cluster electrodes and variable lengths from 10 to 25 cm and can be deployed into star- or umbrella-shaped arrays. Absolute temperature for each device ranges from 15 to 125 °C. Peak power in currently available generators ranges from 150 to 250 W.

Procedure

- This procedure is usually performed under conscious sedation and local anesthesia but may also be performed under general anesthesia with standard cardiac, oxygen, and pressure monitoring.
- Under CT or US guidance, the target lesions are identified.
- Radiofrequency ablation electrodes are positioned in pre-planned locations within the lesion.
- Selection of single or cluster electrodes is made based on operator clinical experience and size of the target lesion.
- Procedure is initiated, and ablation continues until impedance end-point is reached and device turns off or target temperature is reached after gradual increase in generator output power over a 12-min period.
- The targeted ablative margin is 0.5–1 cm beyond the borders of the tumor.

Applications of RFA

Pulmonary Malignancy
- RFA can be used to treat primary lung cancers or metastatic lesions in patients who are nonsurgical candidates, provided that each lesion is smaller or equal to 4 cm in diameter, with a maximum of three lesions per lung in a single patient evaluation.
- Contraindications: Extensive spread of disease, tumor adjacent to major pulmonary vasculature, acute illness, uncorrectable coagulopathy, severe cardiopulmonary disease.
- Complications: pain or paresthesia at puncture site, pneumothorax, pleural effusion, hemothorax, pneumonia, pulmonary abscess, hemoptysis, and chest pain.
- Local recurrence rate of pulmonary tumors after RFA has been documented to range from 3% to 38% with a 3-year survival rate of 15–46% [25].

Hepatic Malignancy
- RFA is well indicated for unresectable early-stage hepatocellular carcinomas and metastatic hepatic lesions, provided that the lesions are smaller or equal to 4 cm in diameter, with a maximum of three hepatic lesions at patient presentation.
- Contraindications: extensive spread of disease, tumor adjacent to major vasculature, acute illness, uncorrectable coagulopathy, impaired liver function (particularly with ascites), tumor abutting major hepatic duct or main biliary duct, intrahepatic bile duct dilatation, and bilioenteric anastomoses.
- Complications: pain or paresthesia at puncture site, subcapsular hematoma, bowel perforation, abscess, hemothorax, tumor seeding, and bile duct injury.
- Local control rates in the liver have been reported at 90% for large tumors (>3 cm), and complete ablation rates have been reported ranging from 91 to 100% [22].
- Three-year survival for patients with HCC treated with RFA ranges from 50 to 91% depending on the study population [22].

Renal Malignancy
- RFA is indicated in renal cell carcinoma patients with biopsy-proven T1a N0 M0 disease, where both surgery and active surveillance are contraindicated. Lesions can be up to 4 cm in diameter, with up to three tumors per presentation.
- Contraindications: Extensive spread of disease, tumor adjacent to major vasculature, acute illness, uncorrectable coagulopathy.
- Complications: pain or paresthesia at puncture site, subcapsular hemorrhage, tumor tract seeding, urethral injury, neuropathic pain along lumbar plexus, and bowel perforation.
- Ablation success rate documented on CT scan for renal tumors has been reported to range from 69% to 100% [23]. A comparison of impedance-based and temperature-based control systems for local control of renal tumors showed no differences in clinical outcomes including clinical efficacy, renal function, and local recurrence [23].

Osteoid Osteoma and Bone Metastases

- RFA is established as the primary therapy for osteoid osteoma, which is a small, painful, benign bone lesion [26]. RFA is also indicated for palliative pain relief in patients with painful osseous lesions who are poor candidates for or have failed standard therapy (radiation, opioid, analgesia), provided that there is no systemic spread of disease [27].
- Contraindications: lesions in the spinal vertebra within 1 cm of neural elements, tumors abutting hollow viscera or neural elements, hypervascular lesions, lesions over 3–4 cm, and risk of fracture in weight-bearing bones [27, 28].
- Complications: pain or paresthesia at puncture site, neural injury, skeletal fracture, and thermal skin burns.

Microwave Ablation

MWA is a thermal ablative technique, whereby tissue heating is caused by water molecule vibrations due to an oscillating electromagnetic field emitted by a microwave antenna. Unlike RFA, MWA does not depend on the electrical conductivity, tissue impedance, or thermal conductivity of tissue. The goal of MWA is to cause coagulation necrosis leading to subsequent cell death similar to RFA. MWA generates heat within a larger heating zone reaching higher temperatures over shorter periods of time than RFA, leading to more uniform zone of necrosis. Like RFA, MWA is less effective in tumors adjacent or near to large vessels due to heat-sink effect; however, this effect is less pronounced in MWA. A 1.0 cm ablation margin is targeted around the tumor with this technique [2, 12, 23, 29–35].

MWA is currently being assessed and evaluated as a viable treatment or palliation technique in hepatic malignancy, pulmonary malignancy, and renal and bone malignancy. The goal of MWA is local tumor control and prolonged survival similar to RFA. Complete ablation is characterized by a non-enhancing region in the location of the tumor and ablative margin on contrast-enhanced imaging (Fig. 10.3).

Device and Technique

The MWA device consists of a microwave generator, power distribution system, and microwave antennae. The microwave generator generates oscillating electromagnetic fields at frequencies greater than 900 MHz (usually 915 MHz) leading to alteration in the rotation of water molecules causing frictional heat production. MWA probes used are primarily 14.5 gauge with active tip lengths of 1.6 or 3.7 cm and a total length of 12, 17, or 22 cm. The probes can be used alone in conjunction with up to two additional probes in order to ablate larger tumors.

Ablation of tumors larger than 2 cm requires multiple microwave antennae placed in the tumor spaced appropriately in order to ensure complete ablation.

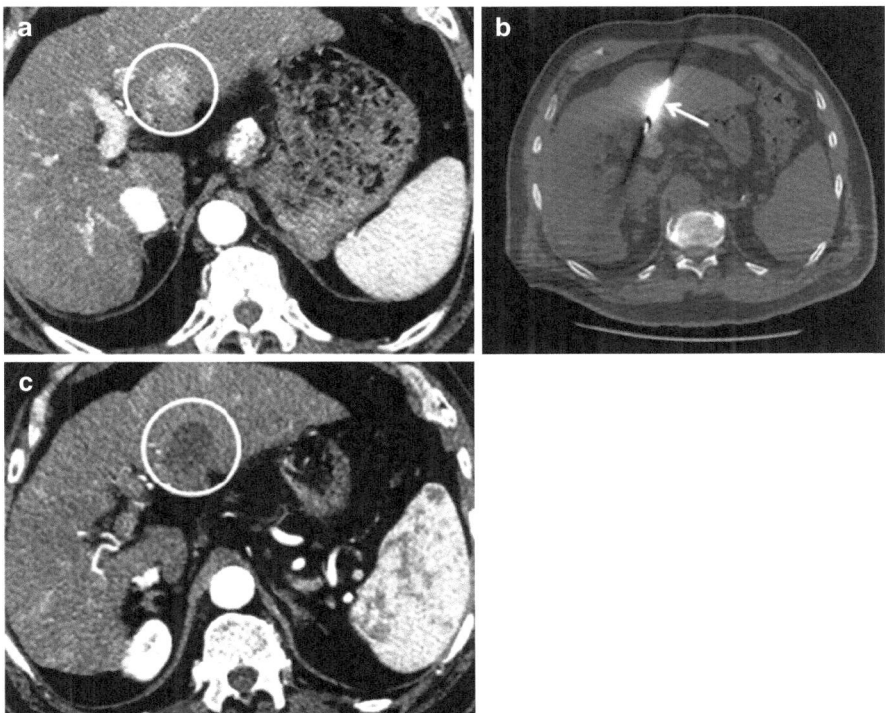

Fig. 10.3 HCC in the left lobe of the liver on an (**a**) arterial-phase contrast CT, (**b**) with MWA needle in position prior to ablation and (**c**) post-ablation arterial-phase contrast CT with a characteristic non-enhancing region suggestive of complete ablation

Procedure

The procedure for MWA is similar to RFA with differences in position of antennae placement and treatment time.

- This procedure is usually performed under conscious sedation and local anesthetic but may also be performed under general anesthesia with standard cardiac, oxygen, and pressure monitoring.
- Under CT or US guidance, the target lesions are identified, and microwave antennae are positioned within the lesion.
- Positioning of the antennae is based on the size of the tumor, the active tip lengths of the probes used, and the required ablative margin.
- MWA is conducted at a power of 45 W for 7–10 min for each ablation area.
- The total ablation time depends on the number of antenna positions required.

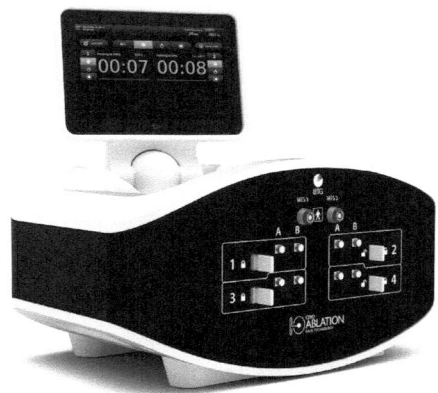

Applications of MWA

Pulmonary Malignancy
- Indications include early-stage primary lung cancer or small number of pulmonary metastases (less than 5) in accessible locations. Pulmonary MWA ablation has also been indicated for palliation of large tumors with invasion into the chest wall causing pain.
- Contraindications: extensive spread of disease, tumor adjacent to major vasculature, acute illness, uncorrectable coagulopathy, severe cardiopulmonary disease.
- Complications: pneumothorax, pleural effusion, hemothorax, pneumonia, pulmonary abscess, hemoptysis, and chest pain.
- Three-year overall survival for patients treated with MWA in the literature was reported to be 24% for pulmonary depending on the study population [34].

Hepatic Malignancy
- MWA ablation is indicated in patients with unresectable primary or metastatic liver cancer with a small number of tumors (usually less than 5).
- Contraindications: extensive spread of disease, tumor adjacent to major structures, acute illness, uncorrectable coagulopathy, liver failure.
- Complications: bile duct stenosis, intractable bleeding, liver abscess, colon perforation, skin burning, and tumor seeding.
- Local 1-year recurrence rate of 2–3% for hepatic malignancies [32].
- Three-year overall survival for patients treated with MWA in the literature was reported to be 72.5% and 30% for primary HCC and hepatic metastases treatment [31, 32].

Renal Malignancy
- MWA ablation is indicated in patients with single, solid renal tumors not eligible for surgery.
- Contraindications: extensive spread of disease, tumors larger than 4 cm, tumor adjacent to major vasculature, acute illness, uncorrectable coagulopathy.
- Complications: subcapsular hemorrhage, tumor tract seeding, urethral injury, and bowel perforation.
- Five-year overall survival for patients treated with MWA for renal tumors was reported to be 67% [35]. Comparison studies of MWA and cryoablation in the setting of small renal masses showed no significant difference in local or metastatic recurrence in lesions treated with MWA compared to cryoablation [36].

Bone Malignancy
- Bone MWA ablation is more effective than RFA and other ablation methods due to the low conductivity and thermal conduction limiting RFA effectiveness. Bone MWA ablation is indicated for treatment of painful osteoid osteomas and metastases [37].

Cryoablation [2, 6, 12, 22, 38, 39]

Cryoablation is a thermal ablative technique, whereby target tissue is rapidly cooled leading to the formation of intracellular ice crystals. The intracellular ice crystals destroy organelles and cell membranes, inducing pore formation and disrupting electrochemical gradient. Tumor death is caused by immediate cell death due to cellular destruction and tonicity changes or initiated apoptosis due to cell homeostasis alteration. Cryoablation also causes small vessel thrombosis resulting in further cell death.

The technique uses a rapid freeze/thaw cycle in order to maximize cellular damage during the procedure. Temperatures reach a minimum of $-130\,^{\circ}$C at the center of the probe and $0\,^{\circ}$C at the boundary of the ablation region defined by the "ice ball" appearance on imaging. Cryoablation is easily visualized with imaging, allowing for better monitoring throughout the procedure, compared to RFA and MWA. Similar to RFA and MWA, a 1.0 cm ablation margin is targeted around the tumor with this technique.

The target outcome for cryoablation, similar to other ablative therapies, is local tumor control. Complete ablation is characterized by a non-enhancing region in the location of the tumor and ablative margin on contrast-enhanced imaging. Intraprocedurally, imaging of the "ice ball" determines effectiveness of probe placement for tumor and margin ablation.

Future work in this area is focused on comparing local recurrence and survival in cryoablation compared to RFA and MWA.

Device and Technique

The cryoablation device consists of a cryoablation system and multiple cryoprobes and temperature gauges. Several types of cryoablation devices are currently available: the ICEFX cryoablation from Boston Sceintific, the PerCryo device (Endocare, Irvine, CA), the Presice device (Yokneam, Israel), and SeedNet and MRI SeedNet systems (Yokneam, Israel).

The PerCryo device has multiple sharp probes available of varying diameters and lengths that can create an ablation zone of 32 × 34 mm to 45 × 64 mm based on the 0 °C boundary. The Presice, SeedNet, and MRI SeedNet systems use an argon-based cooling design for cryotherapy and have an ablation zone ranging from 31 × 36 mm to 40 × 67 mm. All of the systems contain thermal sensors that provide real-time feedback on the temperature.

Procedure

The cryoablation procedure is similar to other thermal ablative therapies, with changes due to differences in ablation volume and probe used.

- This procedure is usually performed under mild to moderate sedation and local anesthetic.
- Under CT, US, or MR guidance, the targeted lesions are identified, and CryoProbes are placed into the center of the tumor.
- Additional probes are placed if necessary based on tumor volume and planned ablative margin.
- Cryoablation is conducted at a maximum temperature of −20 to −40 °C for each ablation area in order to ensure adequate cell damage and small vessel thrombosis.
- Treatment guidelines for the positioning of CryoProbes as well as the duration of ablation depend on the manufacturer specifications of the device used.

Applications of Cryoablation

Currently, cryoablation is primarily used for renal malignancy with preliminary evidence for hepatic lesions.

Hepatic Malignancy
- Hepatic cryoablation can be used as an alternative to RFA in patients with unresectable primary or metastatic liver cancer with a small number of tumors and preserved proportion of the liver.
- Contraindications: Liver failure, high burden of disease, tumor adjacent to major structures, uncorrectable coagulopathy.
- Complications: hemorrhage due to ice ball fracture, cold injury in adjacent structures, pleural effusion, jaundice, intrahepatic abscess [38].
- The 1-, 3-, and 5-year tumor-free survival rate is comparable to RFA [38].

Renal Malignancy

- Renal cryoablation is indicated in patients with single, solid renal tumors not eligible for surgery similar to RFA and MWA.
- Contraindications: High burden of disease, tumor adjacent to major structures, recent myocardial event, uncorrectable coagulopathy, lesions greater than 4 cm.
- Complications: hemorrhage or vascular injury, hematuria, pulmonary embolus, infection, tumor seeding, skin freeze, and cerebrovascular events.
- Local recurrence following cryoablation for renal malignancy was measured to range from 2% to 4% on mean follow-up time ranging from 6 to 27 months [22].

Pulmonary Malignancy
- Pulmonary cryoablation is being tested for use in lung cancer patients who are not surgical candidates.
- Complications: pneumothorax, pleural effusion, hemothorax, pneumonia, pulmonary abscess, hemoptysis, and chest pain.
- Three-year local recurrence rate following cryoablation for pulmonary malignancy was 20.2% for tumors <15 mm in diameter and 71.4% for tumors >15 mm in diameter [39].

High-Intensity Focused Ultrasound

High-intensity focused ultrasound (HIFU) is a minimally invasive, non-ionizing ablation technique that uses ultrasound beams to heat tumor tissue and induce coagulation necrosis. Although the intensity of the beam used for HIFU is 100–1000 times greater than that of diagnostic ultrasound, the beam can pass through overlying structures without causing harm, ablating tissue only at its focal point. In addition to temperature-based ablation, HIFU also delivers mechanical shock to target tissue, by the effect of cavitation. When the ultrasound waves hit liquid, they can cause rapid expansion and collapse of microbubbles, sending damaging shock waves throughout the tissue.

The precision of the ultrasound energy delivery is affected by the distance to the target; therefore HIFU is used mainly for more superficial organs, such as the prostate and uterus. HIFU cannot be used over the bone due to its high density nor over areas of respiration or bowel loops as this affects beam precision.

The noninvasive nature of HIFU, along with its low complication rate and avoidance of ionizing radiation, makes HIFU an attractive alternative to other more radical treatments. This technology has proved promising in many clinical trials and has been utilized in the treatment of various cancers, although indications for routine use and comparisons of efficacy against other treatment modalities still need to be further evaluated.

Device and Technique

HIFU uses a high-power piezoelectric or piezoceramic transducer to focus the ultrasound beams onto a single three-dimensional point, which is typically 1–3 mm in diameter and 10 mm in length [40]. The goal is to heat the target tissues to 60–95 °C for at least 1 s to induce coagulation necrosis. Temperatures above 95 °C should be avoided, as it can produce unpredictable boiling effects.

Lenses and reflectors are often used to focus the ultrasound beam, but recently, phased array transducer systems have been developed, which allow for greater beam control since each part of the ultrasound transducer is supplied by a different electrical signal [41].

The procedure must also be image-guided, either with MRI or diagnostic ultrasound, to ensure that the therapeutic ultrasound beams are focused to a precise target. MRI has a higher resolution and allows for precise monitoring with thermometric maps; however ultrasound is more convenient and portable [40].

HIFU can be applied to larger target areas by performing repeated adjacent ablations. However, ablation of larger regions is time-consuming since the beam must be refocused several times to cover the entire target area and the tissue must be given time to cool adequately between each round of ablation.

Procedure

- The ultrasound transducer can be applied extracorporeally or through a body cavity, such as the rectum or urethra.
- Air-filled areas should be avoided since they affect precision—areas of respiration and bowel loops should not be within the path of the beam.
- Procedure can be performed under epidural, general, spinal, or intravenous anesthesia.
- Chilled, degassed water is streamed over the transducer to cool the surrounding tissues and reduce contact with air.
- The ablated volume is monitored throughout the procedure with MRI or diagnostic ultrasound—MRI does this more accurately with thermometric maps, while ultrasound detects gray scale changes.
- Post-treatment, the surrounding structures (such as skin, bladder, rectum, vagina) are cooled with normal saline solution, and an MRI can be performed to confirm the ablated region.

Applications of HIFU

Uterine Fibroids
- HIFU can be offered as a noninvasive alternative to surgery for patients with symptomatic uterine fibroids up to 10 cm in diameter [42].

- Contraindications: high number of fibroids, absence of an acoustic window (due to scarring or anatomic abnormalities of the bladder and surrounding structures), pregnancy, suspicion of malignancy, acute inflammatory disease.
- Complications: superficial skin burns, abdominal scars, transient pain.
- Five-year overall re-intervention rate was 58.6% in one study [43].

Prostate Cancer
- HIFU is indicated for patients with localized prostate cancer who are not surgical candidates and for those undergoing salvage therapy for recurrent cancer [41].
- Contraindications: calcification in the prostatic tissue (this poses a barrier to beam propagation), pathologic or anatomic conditions that do not permit use of the transducer, metastatic cancer.
- Complications: urinary incontinence, urethral stricture, rectal fistula, hematuria, rectal pain or bleeding.
- Five-year failure-free survival rate (defined as survival with avoidance of metastases, local surgery or radiotherapy, and systemic therapy) is 88% following focal HIFU [44].

Hepatic Malignancy
- HIFU is being evaluated for use with patients with hepatocellular carcinoma or liver metastases up to 8 cm in diameter for whom surgery and radiofrequency ablation are contraindicated [45, 46].
- Contraindications: rib cage malformations, more than three lesions per liver, lesions larger than 8 cm in diameter, bowel loops in the path of sonication.
- Complications: pain, elevated liver enzymes, skin edema, fatigue.
- In one study, most patients (79%) achieved complete response after HIFU treatment [46].

Breast Cancer
- HIFU is being evaluated for the treatment of benign and malignant breast tumors in patients who are not surgical candidates or who prefer breast-conserving management and has shown promising results [47].
- Complications: local mammary edema, minor skin burns and blistering, pectoralis major injury [48].
- In one review, 46% of patients were found to have no residual tumor on histopathology after HIFU ablation, 29% of patients had less than 10% residual tumor, and 23% of patients had 10–90% residual tumor [48].
- Complete tumor ablation has not been reliably reported in smaller studies; therefore large clinical trials have not yet been established.

References

1. Foltz G. Image-guided percutaneous ablation of hepatic malignancies. Semin Intervent Radiol. 2014;31(2):180–6.
2. Hickey R, Vouche M, Sze DY, Hohlastos E, Collins J, Schirmang T, Memon K, Ryu RK, Sato K, Chen R, Gupta R. Cancer concepts and principles: primer for the interventional oncologist—part II. J Vasc Interv Radiol. 2013;24(8):1167–88.
3. Shen A, Zhang H, Tang C, Chen Y, Wang Y, Zhang C, Wu Z. A systematic review of radiofrequency ablation versus percutaneous ethanol injection for small hepatocellular carcinoma up to 3 cm. J Gastroenterol Hepatol. 2013;28(5):793–800.
4. Ahmed M, Brace CL, Lee FT Jr, Goldberg SN. Principles of and advances in percutaneous ablation. Radiology. 2011;258(2):351–69.
5. Lin SM, Lin CJ, Lin CC, Hsu CW, Chen YC. Randomised control trial comparing percutaneous radiofrequency thermal ablation, percutaneous ethanol injection, and percutaneous acetic acid injection to treat hepatocellular carcinoma of 3 cm or less. Gut. 2005;54(8):1151–6.
6. Smith KA, Kim HS. Interventional radiology and image-guided medicine: interventional oncology. Semin Oncol. 2011;38(1):151–62.
7. Monchik JM, Donatini G, Iannuccilli J, Dupuy DE. Radiofrequency ablation and percutaneous ethanol injection treatment for recurrent local and distant well-differentiated thyroid carcinoma. Ann Surg. 2006;244(2):296–304.
8. Fukumoto K, Kojima T, Tomonari H, Kontani K, Murai S, Tsujimoto F. Ethanol injection sclerotherapy for Baker's cyst, thyroglossal duct cyst, and branchial cleft cyst. Ann Plast Surg. 1994;33(6):615–9.
9. Nixon IJ, Angelos P, Shaha AR, Rinaldo A, Williams MD, Ferlito A. Image-guided chemical and thermal ablations for thyroid disease: review of efficacy and complications. Head Neck. 2018;40(9):2103–15.
10. Aycock KN, Davalos RV. Irreversible electroporation: background, theory, and review of recent developments in clinical oncology. Bioelectricity. 2019;1(4):214–34.
11. Philips P, Hays D, Martin RCG. Irreversible electroporation ablation (IRE) of unresectable soft tissue tumors: learning curve evaluation in the first 150 patients treated. PLoS One. 2013;8(11):1–9.
12. Saldanha DF, Khiatani VL, Carrillo TC, et al. Current tumor ablation technologies: basic science and device review. Semin Intervent Radiol. 2010;27(3):247–54.
13. Lee EW, Thai S, Kee ST. Irreversible electroporation: a novel image-guided cancer therapy. Gut Liver. 2010;4(Suppl 1):S99–104.
14. Vlaisavljevich E, Maxwell A, Mancia L, Johnsen E, Cain C, Xu Z. Visualizing the histotripsy process: bubble cloud–cancer cell interactions in a tissue-mimicking environment. Ultrasound Med Biol. 2016;42(10):2466–77.
15. Allen SP, Hall TL, Cain CA, Hernandez-Garcia L. Controlling cavitation-based image contrast in focused ultrasound histotripsy surgery. Magn Reson Med. 2015;73(1):204–13.
16. Murad HY, Yu H, Luo D, Bortz EP, Halliburton GM, Sholl AB, Khismatullin DB. Mechanochemical disruption suppresses metastatic phenotype and pushes prostate cancer cells toward apoptosis. Mol Cancer Res. 2019;17(5):1087–101.
17. van Eekeren RR, Boersma D, Holewijn S, Vahl A, de Vries JP, Zeebregts CJ, Reijnen MM. Mechanochemical endovenous ablation versus RADiOfriqueNcy ablation in the treatment of primary great saphenous vein incompetence (MARADONA): study protocol for a randomized controlled trial. Trials. 2014;15(1):1–7.
18. Murad HY, Bortz EP, Yu H, Luo D, Halliburton GM, Sholl AB, Khismatullin DB. Phenotypic alterations in liver cancer cells induced by mechanochemical disruption. Sci Rep. 2019;9(1):1–3.
19. Kunzli BM, Abitabile P, Maurer CA. Radiofrequency ablation of liver tumors: actual limitations and potential solutions in the future. World J Hepatol. 2011;3(1):8–14.

20. Gervais DA, McGovern FJ, Arellano RS, McDougal WS, Mueller PR. Radiofrequency ablation of renal cell carcinoma: part I, indications, results, and role in patient management over a 6-year period and ablation of 100 tumors. AJR Am J Roentgenol. 2005;185:64–71.
21. Crocetti L, de Baere T, Lencioni R. Quality improvement guidelines for radiofrequency ablation of liver tumors. Cardiovasc Intervent Radiol. 2010;33:11–7.
22. Kwan KG, Matsumoto ED. Radiofrequency ablation and cryoablation of renal tumors. Curr Oncol. 2007;14(1):34–8.
23. Izzo F, Granata V, Grassi R, Fusco R, Palaia R, Delrio P, et al. Radiofrequency ablation and MWA in liver tumours: an update. Oncologist. 2019;24:e990–e1005.
24. Modabber M, Martin J, Athreya S. Thermal versus impedance-based ablation of renal cell carcinoma: a meta-analysis. Cardiovasc Intervent Radiol. 2014;37:176–85.
25. Zhu JC, Yan TD, Morris DL. A systematic review of radiofrequency ablation for lung tumors. Ann Surg Oncol. 2008;15(6):1765–74.
26. Kurup AN, Callstrom MR. Image-guided percutaneous ablation of bone and soft-tissue tumors. Semin Intervent Radiol. 2010;27(3):276–84.
27. Papathanassiou ZG, Megas P, Petsas T, Papachristou DJ, Nilas J, Siablis D. Osteoid osteoma: diagnosis and treatment. Orthopedics. 2008;31(11):1118.
28. Tam A, Ahrar K. Palliative interventions for pain in cancer patients. Semin Intervent Radiol. 2007;24(4):419–29.
29. Sheu YR, Hong K. Percutaneous lung tumor ablation. Tech Vasc Interv Radiol. 2013;16(4):239–52.
30. Lubner MG, Brace CL, Hinshaw JL, Lee FT Jr. Microwave tumor ablation: mechanism of action, clinical results and devices. J Vasc Interv Radiol. 2010;21(8 Suppl):S192–203.
31. Liang P, Yu J, Lu MD, et al. Practice guidelines for ultrasound-guided percutaneous microwave ablation for hepatic malignancy. World J Gastroenterol. 2013;19(33):5430–8.
32. Martin RC, Scoggins CR, McMasters KM. Safety and efficacy of microwave ablation of hepatic tumors: a prospective review of a 5-year experience. Ann Surg Oncol. 2010;17(1):171–8.
33. Castle SM, Salas N, Leveillee RJ. Initial experience using microwave ablation therapy for renal tumor treatment: 18-month follow-up. Urology. 2011;77(4):792–7.
34. Lu Q, Cao W, Huang L, et al. CT-guided percutaneous microwave ablation of pulmonary malignancies: results in 69 cases. World J Surg Oncol. 2012;10:80.
35. Yu J, Liang P, Yu XL, et al. US-guided percutaneous microwave ablation versus open radical nephrectomy for small renal cell carcinoma: intermediate-term results. Radiology. 2014;270(3):880–7.
36. Martin J, Athreya S. Meta-analysis of cryoablation versus microwave ablation for small renal masses: is there a difference in outcome? Diagn Interv Radiol. 2013;19:501–7.
37. Goetz MP, Callstrom MR, Charboneau JW, et al. Percutaneous image-guided radiofrequency ablation of painful metastases involving bone: a multicenter study. J Clin Oncol. 2004;22(3):300–6.
38. Wang C, Wang H, Yang W, Hu K, Xie H, Hu KQ, et al. Multicenter randomized controlled trial of percutaneous cryoablation versus radiofrequency ablation in hepatocellular carcinoma. Hepatology. 2015;61(5):1579–90.
39. Yamauchi Y, Izumi Y, Kawamura M, et al. Percutaneous cryoablation of pulmonary metastases from colorectal cancer. PLoS One. 2011;6(11):e27086.
40. Izadifar Z, Izadifar Z, Chapman D, Babyn P. An introduction to high intensity focused ultrasound: systematic review on principles, devices, and clinical applications. J Clin Med. 2020;9(2):460.
41. Napoli A, Alfieri G, Scipione R, Leonardi A, Fierro D, Panebianco V, et al. High-intensity focused ultrasound for prostate cancer. Expert Rev Med Devices. 2020;17(3):427–33.
42. Masciocchi C, Arrigoni F, Ferrari F, Giordano AV, Iafrate S, Capretti I, et al. Uterine fibroid therapy using interventional radiology mini-invasive treatments: current perspective. Med Oncol. 2017;34(4):52.

43. Quinn SD, Vedelago J, Gedroyc W, Regan L. Safety and five-year re-intervention following magnetic resonance-guided focused ultrasound (MRgFUS) for uterine fibroids. Eur J Obstet Gynecol Reprod Biol. 2014;182:247–51.
44. Guillaumier S, Peters M, Arya M, Afzal N, Charman S, Dudderidge T, et al. A multicentre study of 5-year outcomes following focal therapy in treating clinically significant nonmetastatic prostate cancer. Eur Urol. 2018;74(4):422–9.
45. Zhang L, Zhu H, Jin C, Zhou K, Li K, Su H, et al. High-intensity focused ultrasound (HIFU): effective and safe therapy for hepatocellular carcinoma adjacent to major hepatic veins. Eur Radiol. 2008;19:437–45.
46. Yang T, Ng DM, Du N, He N, Dai X, Chen P, et al. HIFU for the treatment of difficult colorectal cancer with unsuitable indications for resection and radiofrequency ablation: a phase I clinical trial. Surg Endosc. 2021;35:2306–15.
47. Peek MCL, Ahmed M, Napoli A, ten Haken B, McWilliams S, Usiskin SI, et al. Systematic review of high-intensity focused ultrasound ablation in the treatment of breast cancer. Br J Surg. 2015;102(8):873–82.
48. Feril LB, Fernan RL, Tachibana K. High-intensity focused ultrasound in the treatment of breast cancer. Curr Med Chem. 2021;28(25):5179–88.

Part III
Common Interventional Radiology Procedures

Chapter 11
Thoracic Interventional Radiology

Ruqqiyah Rana and Lazar Milovanovic

Percutaneous Thoracic Biopsy

PTB has become common in the field of thoracic radiology and provides a minimally invasive method by which lung, mediastinal, or pleural tissue can be collected in order to diagnose thoracic pathologies. The goal of the procedure is to obtain enough tissue or cells required to meet diagnostic needs for pathologic assessment. PTB is now primarily done under computed tomography (CT) but can also be done under fluoroscopy and ultrasound guidance for pleural- based lesions [1]. Imaging modality of choice for procedural guidance depends on lesion location and operator preference [1]. Biopsy can be done using fine needle aspiration (FNA) for cytology or core needle biopsy (CNB) for histopathologic tissue analysis [2]. Studies have shown the accuracy of diagnosis for thoracic lesions using coaxial 18-gauge core needle biopsy to be around 97%, with a complication rate of around 19% [3].

Percutaneous Transthoracic Lung Biopsy

Indications

Indications for PTLB [1, 2, 4, 5] are based on the SIR percutaneous needle biopsy guidelines developed by Gupta et al. in 2010 and the British Thoracic Society (BTS) guidelines developed by Manhire et al. in 2003 and may include [4, 6]:

- Targeted focal lung lesions
- Lesion or nodule inaccessible via bronchoscopy

R. Rana (✉) · L. Milovanovic
Michael G. DeGroote School of Medicine, McMaster University, Hamilton, ON, Canada
e-mail: ruqqiyah.rana@medportal.ca; lazar.milovanovic@medportal.ca

- Lesions with inconclusive/nondiagnostic bronchoscopic biopsy results
- Multiple nodules in patient with no known malignancy, with prolonged remission or with more than one primary malignancy diagnosis
- Focal infiltrates persisting over time with no diagnosis based on other investigations
- Mass/lesion present in hilum
- Collection of tissue for microbiologic analysis in cases of suspected or known infection
- Diagnosis and characterization of diffuse parenchymal diseases

Contraindications

All contraindications for this procedure are relative, and the risks of the procedure should be weighed against the benefit of performing it prior to making a decision to biopsy [1]:

- Increased risk of bleeding or current use of anticoagulation therapy: platelet count <50,000/mL and aPTT ratio or PT ratio >1.5
- Emphysema
- Presence of bullae
- Impaired lung function
- Prior pneumonectomy
- Pulmonary hypertension
- Lack of patient cooperation
- Predicted forced expiratory volume in 1 s (FEV1) of less than 35% [4]

Pre-procedural Assessment and Imaging

Pre-procedural imaging (primarily chest radiographs, CT scans, or PET/CT) is assessed to locate the lesion to be biopsied, determine appropriateness of biopsy, and plan the access approach to the lesion in order to perform the procedure [4]. Coagulation indices including prothrombin time (PT), activated partial thromboplastin time (aPTT), and platelet count are determined. Oral anticoagulants should be managed (stopped or left unchanged) based on anticoagulation use guidelines outlined in Chap. 5 [1, 4].

Imaging Guidance

PTB can be completed under CT, ultrasound, or fluoroscopic guidance. Ultrasound is the least expensive, safest, and fastest method for image guidance but can only be used when lesions are located peripherally and contact the pleura (less than 30% of

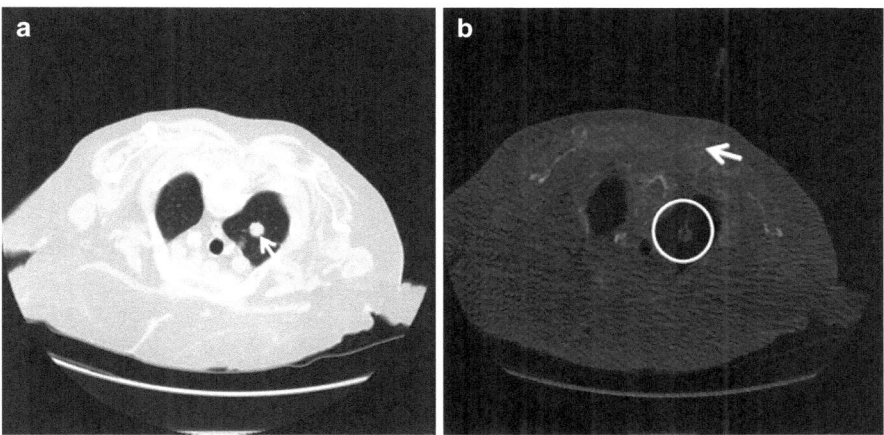

Fig. 11.1 Axial CT of thorax with (**a**) focal lung lesion (*solid arrow*) and (**b**) biopsy needle (*solid line*) placed under CT guidance transthoracically into lesion (*circle*)

all thoracic lesions) [1]. CT guidance provides axial imaging slices and can be used for lesions unsuitable for ultrasound guidance (Fig. 11.1) [1]. In some cases, such as highly mobile lesions, fluoroscopy, or CT fluoroscopy may be useful for real-time visualization of needle position [2].

Procedure

- PTB can be performed under local anesthetic where possible without sedation [4].
- The patient should be positioned in order to minimize the length of aerated lung traversed.
- A radiopaque grid is used to map the optimal access point.
- After administration of local anesthetic, with or without sedation, a small incision is made using a scalpel blade.
- At this point, a biopsy coaxial needle, with needle size selected by the interventional radiologist based on the lesion size and depth, is introduced into the target tissue.
- A biopsy gun loaded with a coaxial biopsy needle (usually 20 gauge) is then carefully introduced and activated.
- Two or three tissue or cell samples are collected and sent for diagnostic analysis and sample characterization.

Complications

Reported complications of PTB include pneumothorax, tumor implantation, air embolism, subcutaneous emphysema, mediastinal emphysema, empyema, bronchopleural fistula, and bleeding complications including hemoptysis, hemothorax, arteriobronchial fistula, and pulmonary hemorrhage [6].

Of these complications, the most common are pneumothorax and pulmonary hemorrhage. Estimated mortality from this procedure has been reported between 0.07% and 0.15% [7, 8]. Pneumothorax occurs in 12–45% of cases, and of these cases, 2–15% require chest tube insertion for pneumothorax management [6].

Variability in pneumothorax rates is due to varying patient populations, differences in pneumothorax definition and diagnosis, as well as the type of imaging used in the intra- and post-procedure assessment to characterize pneumothorax. Risk factors for pneumothorax include large biopsy needles used, number of pleural punctures, size and depth of lesion, pre-existing lung disease, lack of patient cooperation, and operator inexperience.

Pulmonary hemorrhage has been reported without hemoptysis in 5–17% of patients and with hemoptysis in 1.25–5% of patients [7, 8]. Risk factors for hemorrhage include increasing lesion depth, long biopsy path, small lesion size, and emphysema.

Core Needle Biopsy Vs. Fine Needle Aspiration

Overall complication rates differ based not only on the factors mentioned above but also on the mode of biopsy: core needle vs. fine aspiration [9]. A meta-analysis looking at over 12,000 procedures found that the overall complication rate for core biopsy is 38.8% and for fine needle aspiration is 24.0%. For FNA, increased needle diameter, decreased size of lesion, and a greater surface area of lung tissue pierced increased the risk of complications [9]. In both core needle biopsy and fine needle aspiration, the rate of minor complications was greater than major complications.

Post-procedure Imaging

Imaging in the post-procedure setting is important for the assessment of immediate and delayed patient complications following lung biopsy, particularly pneumothorax [1]. Upright chest radiographs and chest CT can be used in the post-procedure setting to assess for complications immediately after the procedure is concluded and should be repeated prior to discharge or if patients develop clinical signs of complications.

Outcomes

Reported success rate for thoracic or pulmonary needle biopsy ranges from 77% to 96% [2, 6]. Comparison of CNB and FNA diagnostic accuracy rates across different types of biopsy findings showed comparable diagnostic accuracy for FNA in malignant tumors (85.1% versus 86.7%) and malignant epithelial neoplasms (86.4% vs. 85.2%) with higher diagnostic accuracy in CNB for malignant nonepithelial neoplasms (96% vs. 77%) as well as benign-specific lesions (92% vs. 40%) [2].

Mediastinal Biopsy

Indications and Contraindications

Percutaneous image-guided biopsy of mediastinal lesions is indicated for lesions which are inaccessible to mediastinoscopy or transbronchial biopsy. There are several contraindications to this procedure which are similar to those for percutaneous lung biopsy including [1, 5, 10]:

- Increased risk of bleeding or anticoagulation therapy: platelet count <50,000/ml and aPTT ratio or PT ratio >1.5
- Lack of patient cooperation

The procedure may not be contraindicated in patients with poor lung function due to lower risk of pulmonary complications [1, 5, 10].

Image Guidance and Procedure: Ultrasound Vs. CT

Percutaneous image-guided mediastinal biopsy is done under CT guidance. Ultrasound guidance is primarily for anterior mediastinal lesions and provides real-time feedback on needle positioning and access. The safety and accuracy of sonographically guided interventions in these situations is equivalent to CT and is only 3/4 the cost [11]. Further, sonographic (ultrasound) procedures are especially adept at localizing blood flow and depicting vessels [11]. Nevertheless, multiple approaches can be used depending on patient factors and target lesion location including extrapleural, transpulmonary, or direct mediastinal (parasternal, paravertebral, transsternal, suprasternal, subxiphoid) approaches. Direct mediastinal approaches utilize the extrapleural space medial to the lungs in order to avoid lung and pleural tissue. The most commonly used technique is a coaxial approach utilizing a guide needle positioned near the target lesion and advancement of the biopsy needle through the guide needle to complete tissue collection.

Complications

Complications include [5]:

- Vascular injury
- Esophageal perforation
- Tracheobronchial injury
- Mediastinitis
- Chylothorax
- Pericardial rupture
- Pneumothorax
- Phrenic nerve injury
- Arrhythmias

Post-procedure Imaging

Post-procedure imaging is targeted toward identifying developing complications prior to clinical symptom development. Chest radiograph or, occasionally, CT scan is performed immediately post-procedure and prior to discharge [1].

Percutaneous Drainage of Thoracic Fluid Collections

Image-guided percutaneous aspiration with or without drainage of fluid or air within the thorax is considered a first-line therapy. Image guidance provides improved safety and efficacy of the procedure over blind techniques. Fluid collections can occur in the pleural space, pericardium, lung, or mediastinum. Pleural fluid collections include pleural effusions, empyema, hemothorax, and chylothorax (chyle accumulating in the pleural cavity). Pulmonary fluid collections include abscesses, pneumatocele, and bullae. Mediastinal fluid collections include abscesses, pericardial effusion, and tension pneumomediastinum [1].

Indications

Indications include [1, 12]:

- Pleural effusion: small pleural effusion can be managed conservatively without aspiration or drainage, while large, symptomatic, or malignant pleural effusions require aspiration or drainage (Fig. 11.2).
- Empyema: requires drainage in addition to antibiotic therapy for management.

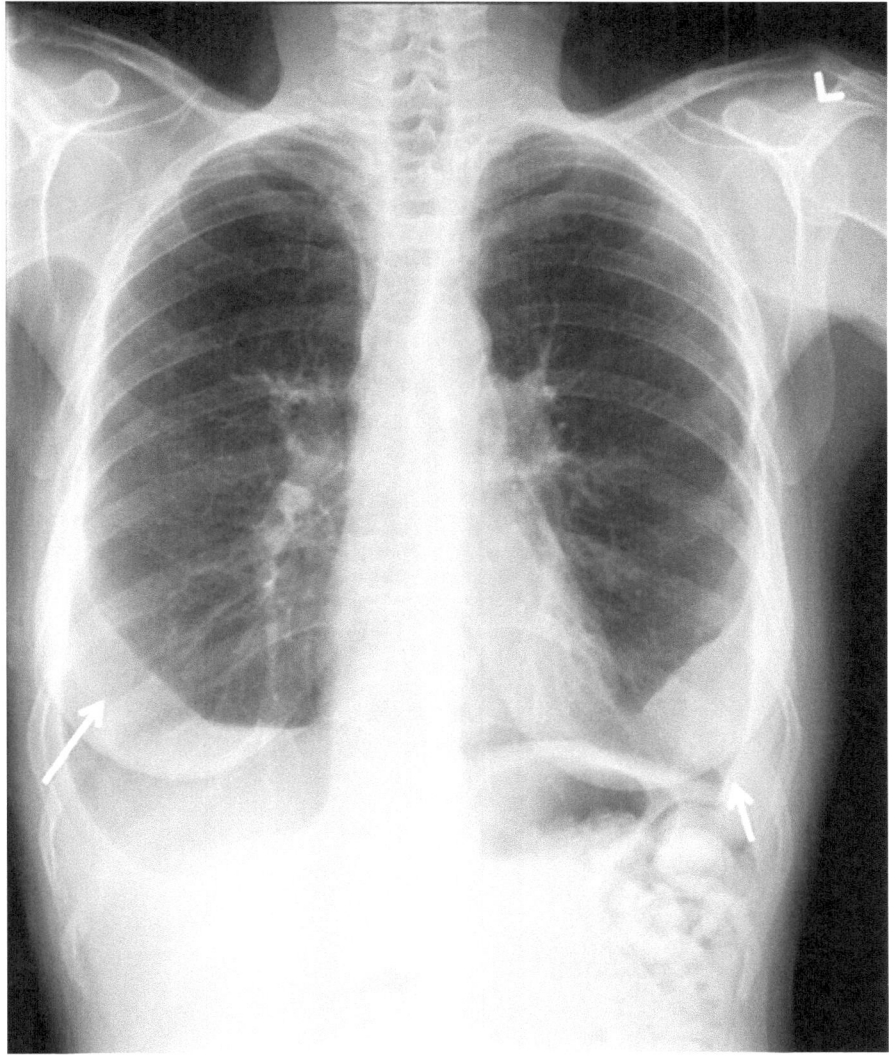

Fig. 11.2 Bilateral pleural effusions, right larger than left (*solid arrows*) on chest radiograph

- Drainage needs to occur early in order to prevent progression of empyema to organized phase. If percutaneous drainage fails, surgical drainage and decortication are the next steps in management.
- Hemothorax: usually occurs in a posttraumatic setting and needs to be drained using large-bore chest tubes. Fibrinolytic agent injection may be required in addition to drainage. Depending on the source of the bleeding, arterial embolization may be required prior to drainage.

- Chylothorax: low-output chylothorax can be managed conservatively using thoracentesis or chest tube drainage until the thoracic duct leak closes, whereas high-output chylothorax will need surgical intervention for thoracic duct leak closure [13].
- Abscesses: may require percutaneous drainage if medical treatment, postural drainage, and bronchoscopic drainage are ineffective (Fig. 11.3).
- Pneumatocele and bullae: drainage is indicated in infected or tension pneumatocele.
- Pericardial effusion: diagnostic pericardiocentesis is indicated if origin is not Known, and therapeutic pericardiocentesis may be considered for symptomatic or large pericardial effusion [14].
- Tension pneumomediastinum: this is an emergency that requires intervention and is primarily managed through mediastinostomy or percutaneous catheter venting under CT guidance.

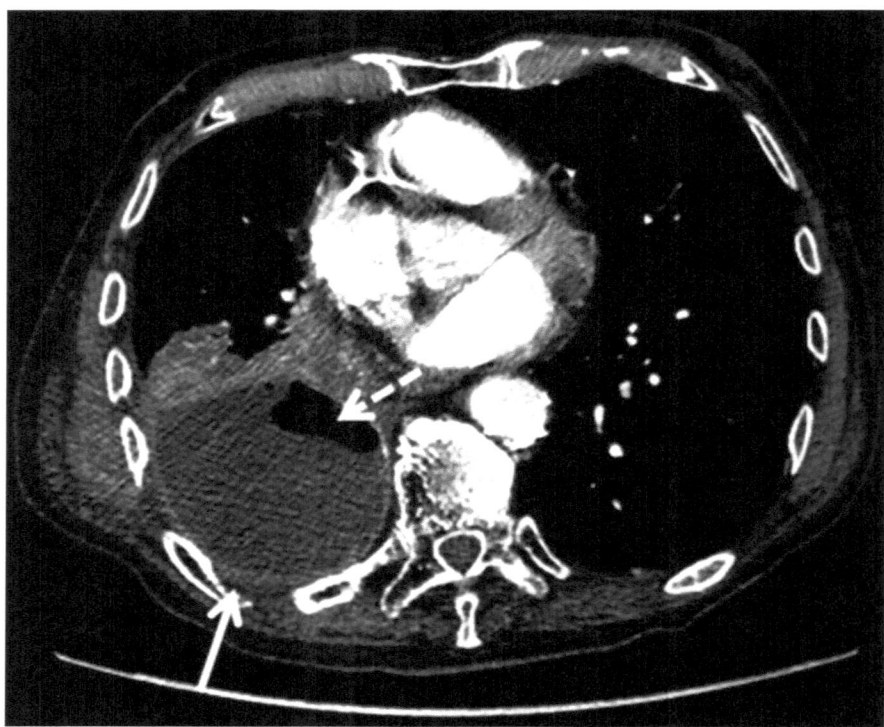

Fig. 11.3 Right lower pleural collection (*solid arrow*) with air-fluid level inside (*dashed arrow*) on axial CT suggestive of abscess

Contraindications

Contraindications include [1, 12]:

- Increased risk of bleeding or anticoagulation therapy: platelet count <50,000/mL and aPTT ratio or PT ratio >1.5
- Uncooperative patients
- Intractable coughing or breathing
- Patients unable to tolerate procedure-induced pneumothorax
- Skin surface infection

Procedure

Percutaneous image-guided fluid drainage and aspiration is primarily done under ultrasound or CT guidance. Ultrasound guidance is preferred for fluid collections located peripherally in the thorax due to real-time guidance, decreased cost, decreased radiation, and ease of use. Aspiration and drainage are primarily done under local anesthetic with sedation in some situations [12].

Complications

Complications include [1, 12]:

- Procedure failure
- Pneumothorax—increased risk when using large-bore needles or aspirating/draining larger quantities of fluid
- Hemorrhage—avoid subcostal approach in order to reduce risk of laceration of intercostal vessels
- Re-expansion pulmonary edema—increased risk of occurrence when lung tissue has been collapsed for a longer duration and a large amount of fluid is drained
- Visceral injury
- Empyema or infection spread following lung abscess drainage

Post-procedure Imaging and Procedural Outcomes

Post-procedure imaging (plain chest X-ray or CT scan) is targeted toward identifying developing complications following the procedure and assessing technical success of the procedure (Fig. 11.4). Procedural outcome is characterized by acute and delayed symptom improvement and reduction in fluid collection volume on imaging [1, 12].

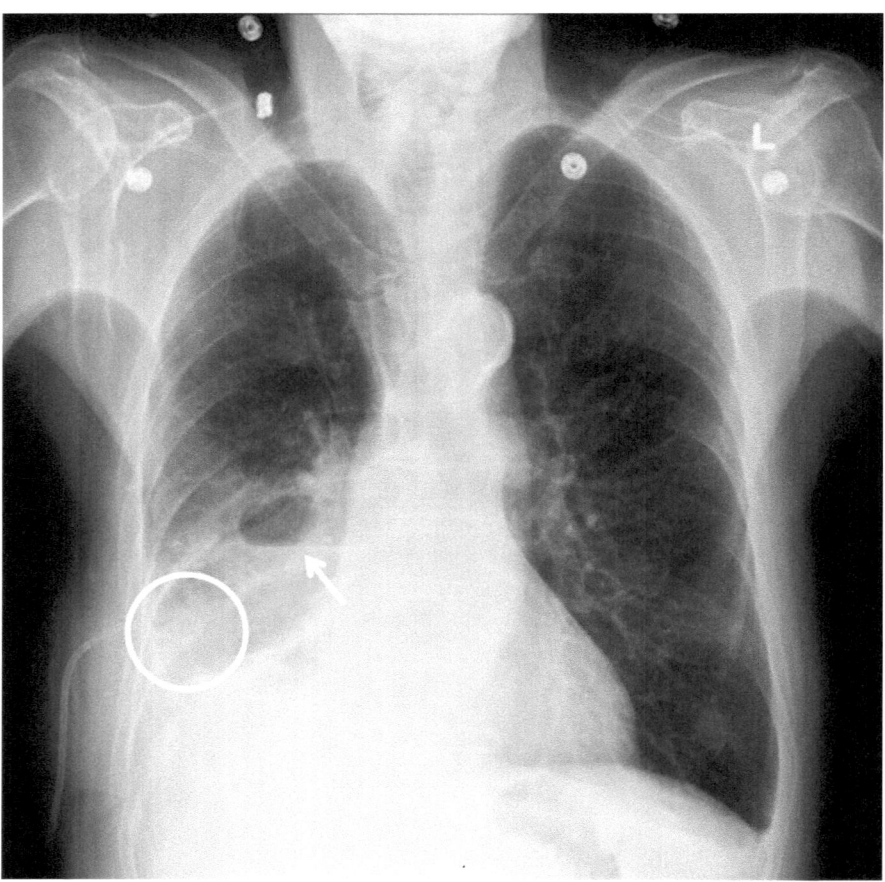

Fig. 11.4 Chest radiograph of patient with a large right-sided complex collection with an air-fluid level (*solid arrow*) and a pig tail catheter in appropriate position (*circle*)

Vascular Interventional Radiology Procedures

There are multiple interventional radiology procedures focusing on pathologies of the thoracic vasculature. These procedures are focused primarily on the treatment of hemoptysis, pulmonary arteriovenous malformations, pseudoaneurysms, and superior vena cava (SVC) obstruction. Common vascular thoracic interventions include bronchial artery embolization for hemoptysis and pulmonary artery arteriovenous malformation (AVM) embolization. Summarized here is the management for hemoptysis using bronchial artery embolization and embolization for pulmonary artery AVMs [1, 12].

Hemoptysis and Bronchial Artery Embolization

Hemoptysis is defined as coughing up blood originating from the lower respiratory tract and can be differentiated into minor (<30 mL), moderate to severe (30–300 mL), and massive (>300 mL) based on the quantity of expectorated blood. Patients with massive hemoptysis (>300 mL per 24 h) have high mortality primarily due to the risk of asphyxiation and aspiration. Bleeding may originate from both small and large lung vessels [1, 12, 15, 16].

Infectious and inflammatory causes of hemoptysis include abscess, chronic bronchitis, bronchiectasis, pneumonia, fungal infections, and tuberculosis. Oncologic causes of hemoptysis include primary or metastatic pulmonary malignancy. Vascular causes of hemoptysis include pulmonary vasculitis, arteriovenous malformations, and pulmonary artery aneurysms. Ninety percent of cases of massive hemoptysis requiring intervention originate from the bronchial arteries [17].

Pre-procedural Imaging and Diagnosis

Bronchoscopy is useful as a first-line diagnostic tool to diagnose active hemorrhage and identify the site of bleeding. Diagnostic imaging modalities for the assessment and characterization of hemoptysis include chest radiographs, CT and CT angiography, and digital subtraction angiography (DSA) [1, 12, 15, 16].

Chest radiography is considered the initial method to evaluate patients with hemoptysis and can help assess focal or diffuse involvement of lung and identify underlying parenchymal and pleural abnormalities but has a very low sensitivity. Bronchoscopy is more effective in localizing the bleeding site in moderate to severe hemoptysis cases compared to mild presentations [1, 12, 15, 16].

Compared to bronchoscopy, CT angiography (CTA) scans are equally effective at characterizing the site of bleeding and are further able to detect neoplasms or bronchiectasis that may be underlying in patients with hemoptysis. CT and CTA provide a method to comprehensively evaluate the lung parenchyma, airways, and thoracic vasculature as well as develop more detailed and accurate maps of the thoracic vasculature than DSA [1, 12, 15, 16].

DSA is indicated in cases where other diagnostic imaging techniques including CTA have been attempted and endovascular treatment has been attempted but was unsuccessful [1, 12, 15, 16].

Active extravasation is observed in only 10.7% of examinations [18]. Abnormal bronchial artery diameter (>3 mm) on angiography in conjunction with bronchoscopic findings and clinical correlation is used in addition to observed extravasation to improve sensitivity and specificity of localization of the bleeding source [18, 19].

Contraindications

Contraindications for this procedure include general contraindications to angiography due to the use of contrast media and angiography for intra-procedural image guidance [1, 12, 15, 16, 19]:

- Uncorrected coagulopathy—this may be due to anticoagulation, vitamin K deficiency, or medical conditions including liver disease, disseminated intravascular coagulation, or platelet deficiency.
- Impaired renal function—the use of radiopaque contrast throughout this procedure leads to risk of contrast-induced nephrotoxicity, and in particular, the patient should not be dehydrated prior to receiving contrast. Patients allergic to contrast media should be treated with steroids and antihistamines prior to the procedure.

Procedure

A brief neurological exam is performed prior to the commencement of the procedure in order to establish a baseline status.

- Under local anesthetic and conscious sedation, a thoracic aortogram is obtained in order to map the bronchial and systemic non-brachial feeding arteries to the bleeding site.
- Common femoral arterial access is the predominant technique for this procedure.
- Brachial artery access can be used in cases of difficult non-bronchial systemic artery contributions [1, 12, 19, 20].
- A reverse-curved or forward-looking 5, 5.5, or 6 French gauge selective catheter is guided through the common femoral artery into the thoracic aorta and the bronchial artery.
- Using the positioned sheath, microcatheters are threaded through for selective bronchial artery access and to reduce the risk of nontarget embolization [21].
- It is important to ensure placement of the catheter beyond the origin of the spinal cord arteries to reduce the risk of spinal cord embolization.
- Embolization materials that can be used include gelatin sponges, polyvinyl alcohol particles 350–500 μm in diameter, and cross-linked gelatin microspheres.

Common Embolization Agents Used

Choosing the appropriate embolization agent in vascular interventional radiology procedures is critical to avoiding unwanted complications and the morbidity and mortality associated with them, such as nontarget embolization [22].

Clinically, these agents can be classified based on the duration of occlusion that they produce; other methods of classification include:

- Physical state
- Autologous nature
- Biosynthetic or synthetic makeup
- Method of embolization (chemical or mechanical)

Common agents include:

- Temporary agents—clot degradation and recanalization within hours to weeks [22]
- Permanent embolic agents—permanent, degradation resistant vessel occlusion [22]

Outcomes

Technical success, defined by complete embolization of bronchial artery on angiography, occurs in more than 90% of interventions (Fig. 11.5). Clinical success post-embolization ranges from 73% to 94% based on post-procedure symptom assessment and clinical follow-up. Clinical failure is usually due to technically inadequate occlusion or poor characterization of bleeding source on initial arteriography. Rate of recurrence of hemoptysis following embolization is very high, ranging from 10% to 55% for longer-term follow-up period up to 46 months and depends on patient factors, technical factors, and underlying etiology. Patients with underlying infectious processes leading to hemoptysis (such as aspergillosis and tuberculosis) are at elevated risk for recurrence of hemoptysis [1, 12, 19–21].

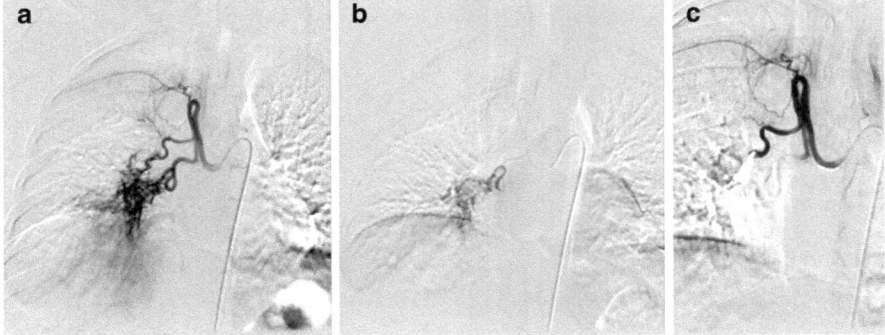

Fig. 11.5 (**a**) Hypertrophied right bronchial artery on angiogram. (**b**) Microcatheter positioned within the right bronchial artery and (**c**) right bronchial artery on angiogram following embolization with angiographic embolization end point visualized

Complications

Patients undergoing this procedure are at risk of angiographic complications including:

- Bleeding/bruising at puncture site
- Puncture site infection
- Allergic reaction to contrast media
- Contrast-induced nephropathy
- Myocardial infarction
- Stroke
- Blood vessel damage
- Death (in rare cases)

In addition, patients undergoing this procedure are at risk of embolization complications including:

- Post-embolization syndrome (pleuritic pain, fever, dysphagia, and leukocytosis lasting 5–7 days).
- Unintentional, nontarget embolization.

Post-embolization syndrome, a condition characterized by pleuritic pain, fever, dysphagia, and leukocytosis, may occur in some patients lasting for 5–7 days. It is managed through symptom relief until resolution. Unintentional, nontarget embolization is the most frequent cause of complications in this procedure including esophageal nontarget embolization leading to transient dysphagia (1–18%). Chest pain is a common complication and may occur in 24–91% of cases. Spinal cord ischemia leading to transverse myelitis is a very severe complication and has been characterized in the literature to occur in 1.4–6.5% of cases [1, 12, 19–21].

Post-procedure Imaging

Additional diagnostic imaging (CXR or CT scan) is completed if patients develop symptoms prior to discharge. Bronchoscopy may be required in follow-up for symptom assessment [1, 12, 19–21, 23].

Pulmonary Arteriovenous Malformations

Pulmonary arteriovenous malformations (AVMs) are direct connections between pulmonary artery branches and corresponding draining pulmonary veins without corresponding capillary beds. Some pulmonary AVMs may be composed of more than one feeding artery and more than one draining vein, may form a plexus, and may be separated or multi-channeled. In pulmonary vasculature, AVMs are primarily congenital but may be acquired secondary to liver cirrhosis, infection, trauma, or malignancy. Approximately 70% of pulmonary arteriovenous malformations occur in patients with hereditary hemorrhagic telangiectasia (HHT). Pulmonary AVMs may increase in size over time and if left untreated can lead to significant morbidity and mortality. Pulmonary AVMs are a potential source of paradoxical emboli due to the right to left shunt created [1, 12, 24].

Indications

Indications include [1, 12, 24]:

- Symptom management—hemoptysis or hemothorax resulting from aneurysmal sac or vessel wall rupture, epistaxis, dyspnea, congestive heart failure, or fulminant respiratory failure
- Hypoxemia management
- Prevention of hemorrhagic and paradoxical embolization complications
- Feeding vessel larger than 3 mm in diameter
- Pulmonary AVM >2 cm in diameter

Untreated pulmonary AVMs have been associated with stroke, transient ischemic attacks, brain abscesses, migraine headaches, and seizures secondary to infected and noninfected material emboli from the right to left shunt [1, 12, 24].

Procedure

Helical CT with 3D reconstruction is used to assess the vasculature supplying the AVM. Selective transcatheter embolization is performed on all of the feeding arteries. Using a common femoral vein approach, a catheter is guided into the pulmonary vasculature and into the AVM supplying vessels. Embolization materials used in this procedure are primarily endoluminal coils, but previous studies have assessed the use of detachable balloons or polyvinyl alcohol [1, 12, 24].

Outcomes

Closure rates of pulmonary AVMs have been documented as 98% in reported literature. Successful embolization of the AVM results in resolution of the right to left shunt. Multiple interventions are necessary in 20–40% of cases. Major issues with failure occur with incomplete characterization of feeding vessels and unrecognized persistent feeding arteries. Recruitment of additional feeding arteries or recanalization of embolized feeding arteries may lead to embolization failure [1, 12, 24].

Post-procedure Imaging: CT

The recanalization rate in post-embolization pulmonary arteriovenous malformation patients can be 3–49% [25]. Post-embolization imaging is recommended in cases of suspected recanalization or embolization failure in individuals with persistent PAVM-like symptoms [25]. For this purpose, CT pulmonary angiography has been recognized as the gold standard; often this will follow conventional follow-up angiography, particularly in the case of patients in whom multiple malformations exist, where all lesions could not be targeted in the same procedure [25].

Complications

Complications include [1, 12, 24]:

- Post-embolization syndrome
- Pulmonary infarction distal to embolization location
- Pleuritic chest pain
- Sepsis
- Retrograde pulmonary embolism
- Paradoxical embolization
- Air embolism—manifesting as angina, bradycardia, transient ischemic episodes, and facial paresthesia

Superior Vena Cava Obstruction

Overview

SVC obstruction (also known as SVC syndrome) is an intrinsic blockage or extrinsic compression of the SVC leading to restriction of venous return to the right atrium (Fig. 11.6). Symptoms related to SVC obstruction may include dyspnea, coughing, and face, neck, upper body, or arm swelling and flushing. More severe symptoms may include tachypnea, cyanosis, dilation of the upper body veins, mental status changes, lethargy, syncope, and fluid collection in the arms and face. Untreated SVC obstruction may result in death. It can be caused by extrinsic primary or metastatic tumors or enlarged lymph nodes compressing the superior vena cava, central venous line-related benign stenosis, and postoperative changes causing

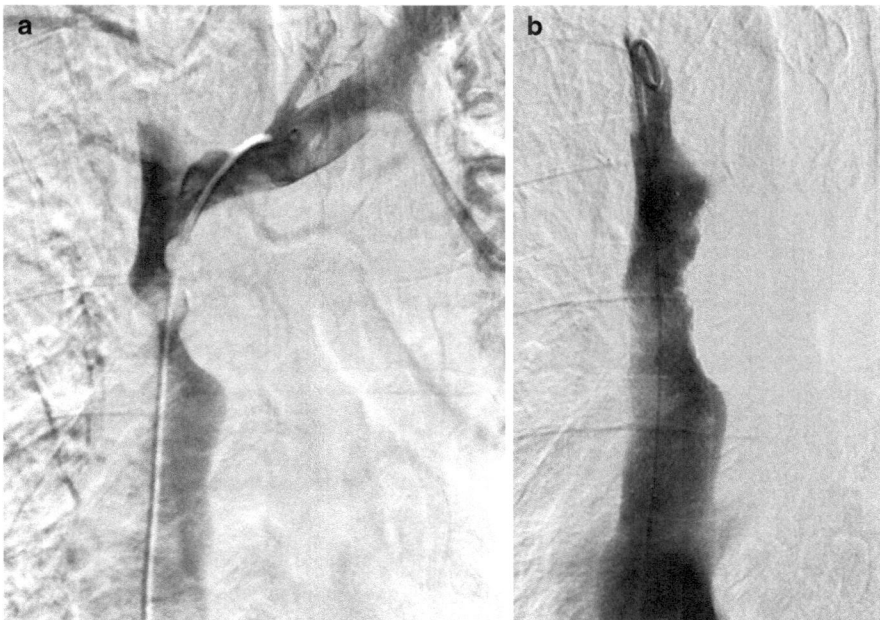

Fig. 11.6 Superior vena cava obstruction with (**a**) catheter placed in the left brachiocephalic vein and (**b**) downstream of the union between the left and right brachiocephalic veins proximal to the heart

stenosis [12, 26]. Medical management of SVC obstruction is done using chemotherapy or radiotherapy. Interventional management of SVC obstruction involves balloon angioplasty and stent placement. Balloon angioplasty and stent placement have become the first-line therapy for SVC obstruction [12, 26].

Pre-procedural Imaging

CT scans of the thorax are used for preliminary imaging, assessment of malignancy including metastases and lymph node involvement, and anatomical changes that may be causing obstruction. After clinical diagnosis has been made, the degree and extent of obstruction is characterized using a venogram at the time of the procedure.

Indications and Contraindications

Stenting has become the first-line therapy for SVC syndrome due to its immediate onset of effect and noninterference with further treatment of thoracic malignancies.

The following must also be considered:

- Patients who have previously received the maximum radiation dose
- Primary and secondary malignant tumors located in the mediastinum

Relative contraindications include:

- Preterminal patient status
- Extensive chronic venous thrombosis
- Endoluminal tumor growth
- Upper limb paralysis
- Inability to undergo fluoroscopy and DSA

Absolute contraindications include unresolvable severe cardiac or coagulation disorders.

Outcomes

Outcome of SVC obstruction stenting and balloon angioplasty is based on post-intervention endoluminal diameter and resolution of clinical symptoms. Overall complete or partial symptom relief was achieved in 68–100% of cases of SVC obstruction due to malignancy across several studies [12]. One in-depth study assessed rates of complete symptom response within 72 h of treatment [26]:

- 66% of patients with headache
- 81% of patients with jugular engorgement
- 76% of patients with collateral venous network on DSA
- 39% of patients with dyspnea and 100% of patients with edema

Average patient survival after stenting was approximately 6 months [26].

Complications

The complication rates of stenting for SVC obstruction are very low but may include [26, 27]:

- Stent migration
- Hemorrhagic complications after local thrombolysis
- Incomplete stent opening
- Thrombus formation
- Pulmonary embolism
- Vascular perforation
- Infection

Acknowledgment We would like to thank Dr. Lazar Milovanovic for his contributions to this chapter (information given on first page of chapter).

References

1. Duncan M, Wijesekera N, Padley S. Interventional radiology of the thorax. Respirology. 2010;15:401–12.
2. Lorenz JM. Updates in percutaneous lung biopsy: new indications, techniques and controversies. Semin Intervent Radiol. 2012;29(4):319–24.
3. Loubeyre P, Copercini M, Dietrich PY. Percutaneous CT-guided multisampling core needle biopsy of thoracic lesions. Am J Roentgenol. 2005;185(5):1294–8.
4. Manhire A, Charig M, Clelland C, Gleeson F, Miller R, Moss H, Pointon K, Richardson C, Sawicka E. Guidelines for radiologically guided lung biopsy. Thorax. 2003;58:920–36.
5. Gupta S, Seaberg K, Wallace MJ, Madoff DC, Morello FA Jr, Ahrar K, Murthy R, Hicks ME. Imaging-guided percutaneous biopsy of mediastinal lesions: different approaches and anatomical considerations. Radiographics. 2005;25:763–88.
6. Gupta S, Wallace MJ, Cardella JF, Kundu S, Miller DL, Rose SC. Quality improvement guidelines for percutaneous needle biopsy. J Vasc Interv Radiol. 2010;21:969–75.
7. Sinner W. Complications of percutaneous thoracic needle aspiration biopsy. Acta Radiol Diagn (Stockh). 1976;17:813–28.
8. Richardson CM, Pointon KS, Manhire AR, Macfarlane JT. Percutaneous lung biopsies: a survey of UK practice based on 5444 biopsies. Br J Radiol. 2002;75(897):731–5.
9. Heerink WJ, de Bock GH, de Jonge GJ, Groen HJ, Vliegenthart R, Oudkerk M. Complication rates of CT-guided transthoracic lung biopsy: meta-analysis. Eur Radiol. 2017;27(1):138–48.
10. Kulkarni S, Kulkarni A, Roy D, Thakur MH. Percutaneous computed tomography-guided core biopsy for the diagnosis of mediastinal masses. Ann Thorac Med. 2008;3(1):13–7.
11. Rubens DJ, Strang JG, Fultz PJ, Gottlieb RH. Sonographic guidance of mediastinal biopsy: an effective alternative to CT guidance. Am J Roentgenol. 1997;169(6):1605–10.
12. Ghaye B, Dondelinger RF. Imaging guided thoracic interventions. Eur Respir J. 2001;17:507–28.
13. Lyon S, Mott N, Koukounaras J, Shoobridge J, Hudson PV. Role of interventional radiology in the management of chylothorax: a review of the current management of high output chylothorax. Cardiovasc Intervent Radiol. 2013;36:599–607.
14. Imazio M, Spodick DH, Brucato A, Trinchero R, Adler Y. Controversial issues in the management of pericardial diseases. Circulation. 2010;121:916–28.
15. Ketai LH, Mohammed TH, Kirsch J, Kanne JP, Chung JH, Donnelly EF, Ginsburg ME, Heitkamp DE, Henry TS, Kazerooni EA, Lorenz JM, McComb BL, Ravenel JG, Saleh AG, Shah RD, Steiner RM, Suh RD, et al. ACR appropriateness criteria hemoptysis. J Thoracic Imaging. 2014;29:W19–22.
16. Larici AR, Franchi P, Occhipinti M, Contegiacomo A, del Ciello A, Calandriello L, Storto ML, Marano R, Bonomo L. Diagnosis and management of hemoptysis. Diagn Interv Radiol. 2014;20:299–309. https://doi.org/10.5152/dir.2014.13426.
17. Bruzzi JF, Remy-Jardin M, Delhaye D, Teisseire A, Khalil C, Remy J. Multi-detector row CT of hemoptysis. Radiographics. 2006;26:3–22.
18. Ramakantan R, Bandekar VG, Gandhi MS, Aulakh BG, Deshmukh HL. Massive hemoptysis due to pulmonary tuberculosis: control with bronchial artery embolization. Radiology. 1996;200(3):691–4.
19. Yoon W, Kim JK, Kim YH, Chung TW, Kang HK. Bronchial and nonbronchial systemic artery embolization for life-threatening hemoptysis: a comprehensive review. Radiographics. 2002;22(6):1395–409.
20. Sopko DR, Smith TP. Bronchial artery embolization for hemoptysis. Semin Intervent Radiol. 2011;28(1):48–62.
21. Burke CT, Mauro MA. Bronchial artery embolization. Semin Intervent Radiol. 2004;21(1):43–8.
22. Medsinge A, Zajko A, Orons P, Amesur N, Santos E. A case-based approach to common embolization agents used in vascular interventional radiology. Am J Roentgenol. 2014;203(4):699–708.

23. De Gregorio MA, Medrano J, Mainar A, Alfonso ER, Rengel M. Endovascular treatment of massive hemoptysis by bronchial artery embolization: short-term and long-term follow-up over a 15-year period. Arch Bronconeumol. 2006;42:49–56.

24. Gossage JR, Kanj G. Pulmonary arteriovenous malformations: a state of the art review. Am J Respir Crit Care Med. 1998;158(2):643–61.

25. Hong J, Lee SY, Cha JG, Lim JK, Park J, Lee J, et al. Pulmonary arteriovenous malformation (PAVM) embolization: prediction of angiographically-confirmed recanalization according to PAVM diameter changes on CT. CVIR Endovasc. 2021;4(1):1–8.

26. Duvnjak S, Andersen PE. Endovascular treatment of superior vena cava syndrome. Int Angiol. 2011;30:458–61.

27. Dahlgren SE, Nordenstrom B. Transthoracic needle biopsy. Chicago: Year Book; 1966.

Chapter 12
Gastrointestinal Interventions

Anne-Sophie Fortier and Prasaanthan Gopee-Ramanan

Radiologically Inserted Gastrostomy (RIG)

Percutaneous endoscopic gastrostomy (PEG) was first performed in 1979 by Gauderer and Ponsky, and the first radiologically inserted gastrostomy (RIG) was performed by Canadian surgeon Preshaw in 1981. Meta-analysis comparing surgical gastrostomy, PEG, and RIG showed success rates of 100%, 95.7%, and 99.2%, respectively [1].

Indications/Contraindications

Indications

- Most common indication is dysphagia which is secondary to head and neck malignancies in 77% of patients and neurological deficits in 18% of patients [2].
- Mucositis and dysphagia occur secondary to radiation therapy of the head and neck.

A.-S. Fortier (✉)
Michael G. DeGroote School of Medicine, Faculty of Health Sciences, McMaster University, Hamilton, ON, Canada
e-mail: annesophie.fortier@medportal.ca

P. Gopee-Ramanan
Department of Radiology, Michael G. DeGroote School of Medicine, Faculty of Health Sciences, McMaster University, Hamilton, ON, Canada
e-mail: prasa.gopee@medportal.ca

© The Author(s), under exclusive license to Springer Nature Switzerland AG 2022
S. Athreya, M. Albahhar (eds.), *Demystifying Interventional Radiology*,
https://doi.org/10.1007/978-3-031-12023-7_12

- For pediatric patients, enteral nutrition can serve as a supplemental feeding route in the context of cystic fibrosis, hydrocephalus, etc.

Contraindications

Contraindications include:

- Uncontrolled/untreated coagulopathy potentiating a risk of internal hemorrhage with INR >1.5 platelet count <50 × 10^9/L.
- Immunosuppression potentiating increased risk of infection should be considered.
- Previous surgery that has interposed colonic bowel or other anatomy, thereby prohibiting interventional access to the stomach.

Procedure

Pre-procedure

- Chart review, coagulation screen, and informed consent procedures are carried out.
- A nasogastric tube (NG) is placed to allow for air dilatation of the stomach; oral effervescent sodium bicarbonate is an alternative to NG tube placement.
- Local anesthesia or conscious sedation can be used.
- Conscious sedation usually consists of midazolam hydrochloride and fentanyl citrate.
- Vital monitoring is then initiated (blood pressure, heart rate, respiratory rate, oxygen saturation).

Procedure

Gastropexy involves the use of 2–4 T-fasteners deployed into the stomach via an 18-gauge needle, which has a reduced risk of initial peritoneal catheterization, gastric leakage, and tube migration and easier replacement of dislodged tubes, thus resulting in fewer repeat RIGs. Skin incision is made overlying the gastric fundus (between T-fasteners if gastropexy performed), and subcutaneous tissues are dissected. The stomach is punctured with an 18-gauge needle, and a stiff guidewire is passed through. The needle is removed, and the tract is dilated in preparation for the catheter—ideally 2-French sizes greater than the catheter diameter. The catheter is advanced (with variation dependent on catheter type and radiologist preference), and intragastric positioning is confirmed via contrast medium injection.

Post-procedure

- The patient should fast for 6 hours before commencement of enteral feeding via feeding gastrostomy.
- Regular flushing following feeding to prevent blockage is recommended. If blocked, warm or carbonated water can be used to remove blockage.

Gastrojejunostomy

A gastrojejunostomy begins similarly to an RIG, but the needle is angled toward the pylorus. A torquable catheter is passed through the pylorus into the duodenum, and a guidewire is advanced past the ligament of Treitz. The tract is then dilated, and a 14–18-French catheter is situated over the guidewire, lying in the proximal small intestine. Contrast medium is injected to confirm positioning by fluoroscopy (Figs. 12.1 and 12.2).

Conversion from RIG to Gastrojejunostomy

If the patient becomes more susceptible to aspiration and reflux, RIG can be converted to a gastrojejunostomy. Rigid sheaths or cannulae can convert the initial RIG angled toward the fundus of the stomach to angle toward the pylorus. If this fails, it may be necessary to create a new tract. Recent literature on minimally invasive techniques for gastrojejunostomy (GJ) tube placement highlight ways to adapt the procedure for different patient populations. In pediatric patients, there is a growing role for laparoscopy and direct visualization of the stomach via endoscope which reduced the patients' radiation exposure [3].

Complications

Complications for RIG and gastrojejunostomy include:

- Infection (aspiration pneumonia, abdominal abscess, cellulitis at the site of incision)
- Hemorrhage
- Tube malposition [2]
- Peritoneal catheterization leading to peritonitis
- Catheter insertion into colon (splenic flexure) leading to diarrhea and gastric bypass of nutrition
- Retrograde migration of the jejunal limb of gastrojejunostomy tube into the stomach and subsequent aspiration and occult gastric feeding [4]
- Catheter occlusion
- Ileus

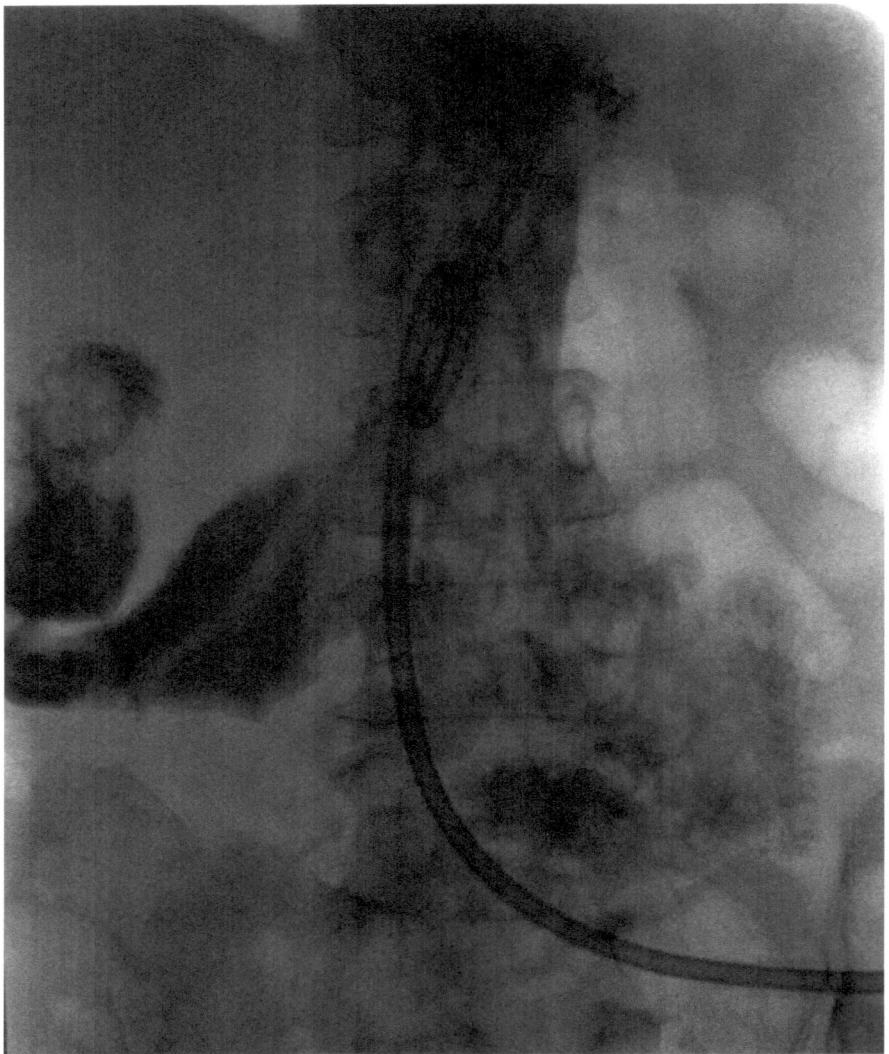

Fig. 12.1 Percutaneous radiology-inserted feeding gastrostomy tube in situ

Esophageal Stenting

Malignant obstruction of the esophagus can result from esophageal carcinoma. Its incidence is increasing in the Western world in the form of adenocarcinoma of the lower third of the esophagus and cardia of the stomach. Dysphagia resulting from extra- or intraluminal obstruction of the esophagus is a cause of significant reduction in quality of life that can be amended via insertion of self-expanding metallic stents (SEMS) or self-expanding plastic stents (SEPS) [5, 6]. SEMS can be inserted under endoscopic or fluoroscopic guidance under conscious sedation (e.g., midazolam 1–5 mg) and oxygen at 2–4 L via nasal prongs.

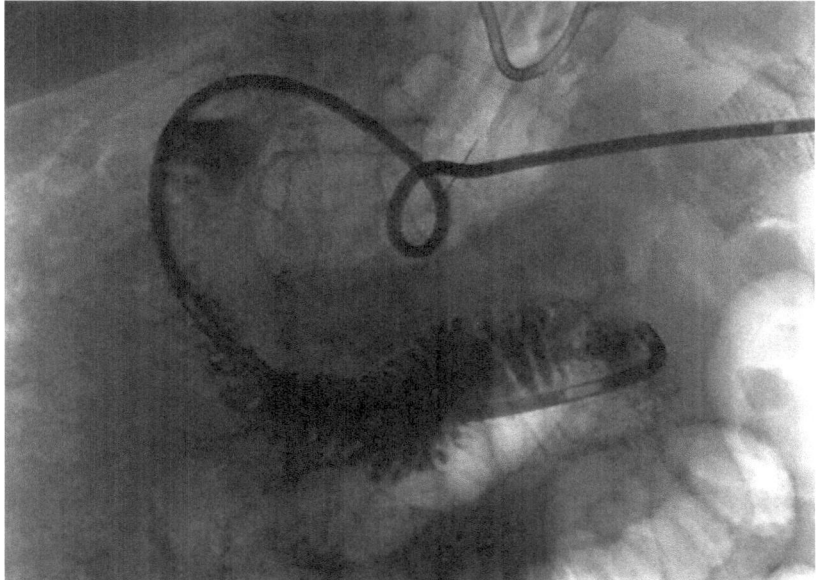

Fig. 12.2   Percutaneous radiology-inserted feeding gastrojejunostomy

For tumors involving the gastroesophageal junction, the patient is placed in a prone position and left lateral position for strictures involving the proximal esophagus. A 5-French catheter with a hydrophilic guidewire is passed into the esophagus until the proximal end of the stricture. The guidewire is then removed, and a 10–15 mL of water-based contrast medium is injected via the catheter. Subsequently, the hydrophilic guidewire is reinserted to help negotiate the stricture and allow for further contrast media to aid in denoting the distal end of the structure. Radiopaque marker placement on the patient's skin can help define stricture length and location [1]. Air insufflation of the stomach prevents the need for excess contrast media to visualize the stomach lining or the tumor. The hydrophilic guidewire is removed and replaced with a stiff guidewire. The catheter is then removed, and the stent deployment unit is inserted. The stent is deployed as to have 2 cm proximally and distally of the proximal and distal ends of the stricture (Fig. 12.3a, b) [1].

Complications

Early complications are uncommon, but delayed complications affect a third of patients, and up to 50% may need re-intervention [7]. Early complications can occur in the first 2–4 weeks and include:

- Chest pain
- Fever
- Bleeding

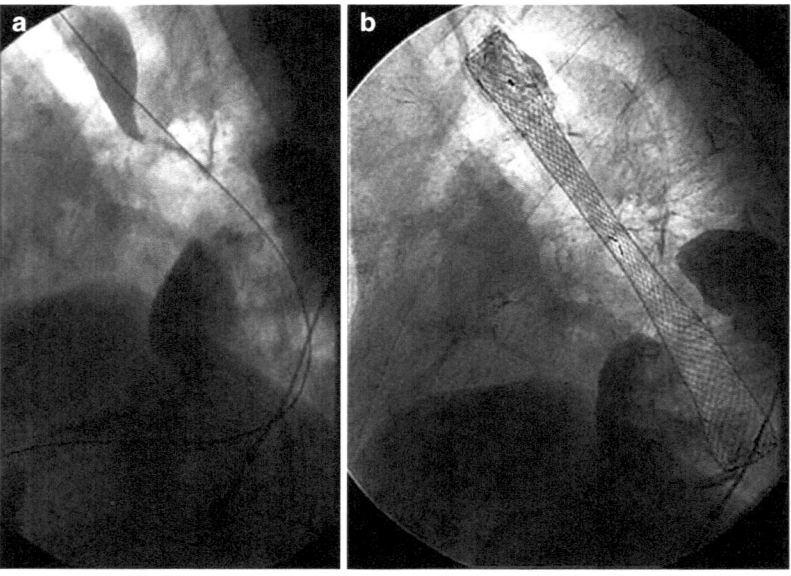

Fig. 12.3 (a) Deployment of esophageal stent under fluoroscopy. (b) Lateral view of esophageal stent in final position

• Gastroesophageal reflux disease (GERD)
• Globus sensation
• Perforation
• Stent migration

Delayed complications occur months after the stent placement and include:

• Tumor ingrowth
• Stent migration
• Stent occlusion
• Development of esophageal fistulae
• Recurrence of strictures [8]

Stent migration is the most common complication between early and delayed categories. Placing an overlapping second stent can rectify partial migration. Fully migrated stents can be endoscopically or surgically removed depending on stent type, risk of perforation, and patient symptoms [6]. The future of esophageal stenting will include stents for benign disease, prevention of GERD post-procedurally, and potential biodegradability [5, 6].

Colonic Stenting

Colonic stenting is an emergency surgery for patients with colonic obstruction, 85% of whom have colorectal cancer, which is associated with significant morbidity and mortality. Both temporary and permanent colostomies have a tremendous impact on the quality of life. Colonic stenting can offer a simpler, durable palliative solution for patients with advanced disease in the left colon proximal to the rectum [9]. It can also be a bridging therapy to surgery as recent literature showed short-term improvements in patient outcomes without long-term disadvantages compared to surgical colon resection [9, 10]. Fluoroscopic-guided colonic stenting is indicated in left-sided lesions more than right-sided. Preparation involves performing a prior water-based contrast enema for lesion localization.

Sedation with midazolam can be considered in high-anxiety or uncooperative patients but is otherwise generally unnecessary. Prophylactic antibiotics in the form of ciprofloxacin and metronidazole can be administered at the physician's discretion as a single dose [9].

The patient is positioned supine or lateral decubitus. A guiding catheter is advanced over a hydrophilic stiff guidewire thereby traversing the obstructed segment of colon. Once the catheter is positioned proximal to the obstruction, water-soluble contrast is again injected to assess the risk of perforation under fluoroscopy. Surface skin radiopaque markers may be used if necessary for localization. Size and delivery system for the stent are decided based upon anatomy visualized and then deployed over the guidewire (Fig. 12.4a–d). Margins of stent coverage should be 2 cm proximal and distal to the respective ends of the obstruction [9].

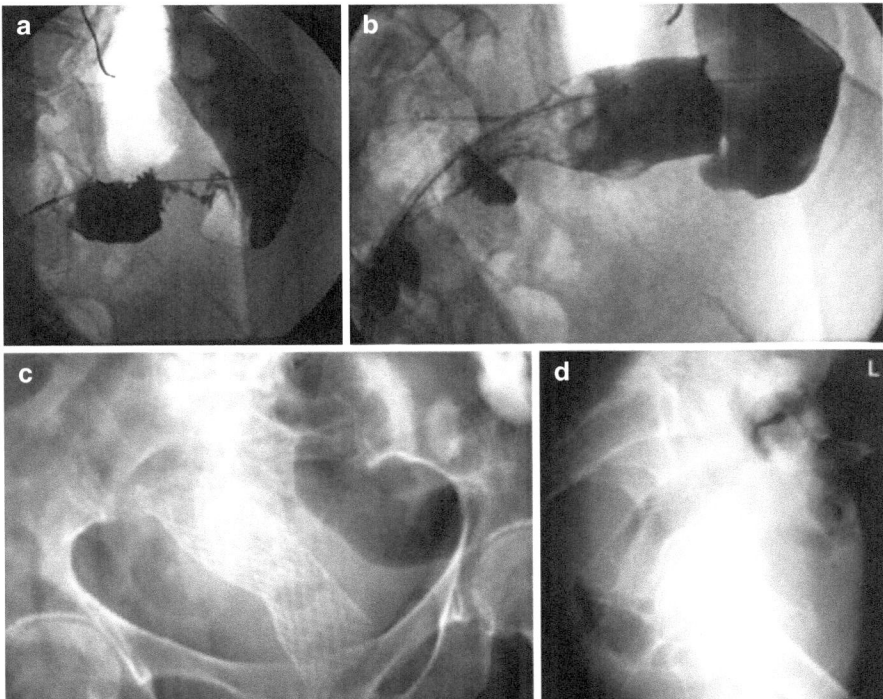

Fig. 12.4 (**a**) Colonic stricture visualized. (**b**) Deployment of colonic stent under fluoroscopy. (**c**) Anteroposterior projection of colonic stent in final position. (**d**) Lateral view of colonic stent in final position

Complications

- Minor complications include mild to moderate rectal bleeding, transient anorectal pain, temporary incontinence, and fecal impaction.
- More severe complications include perforation, re-obstruction, stent migration, and stent fracture [10, 11].

Acknowledgment We would like to thank Dr. Prasaanthan Gopee-Ramanan for his contributions to this chapter (information given on first page of chapter).

References

1. Lyon SM, Pascoe DM. Percutaneous gastrostomy and gastrojejunostomy. Semin Intervent Radiol. 2004;21(3):181–9. https://doi.org/10.1055/s-2004-860876.
2. Dolan RS, Duszak R Jr, Bercu ZL, Martin JG, Newsome J, Kokabi N. Comparing the safety and cost of image-guided percutaneous gastrostomy tube placement in the outpatient versus overnight observation setting in a single-center retrospective study. Acad Radiol. 2021;28(8):1081–5.
3. Gerall C, Mencin AA, DeFazio J, Griggs C, Kabagambe S, Duron V. Primary gastrojejunostomy tube placement using laparoscopy with endoscopic assistance: a novel technique. J Pediatr Surg. 2021;56(2):412–6.
4. Johnson DY, Gallo CJ, Agassi AM, Sag AA, Martin JG, Pabon-Ramos W, et al. Percutaneous gastrojejunostomy tubes: identification of predictors of retrograde jejunal limb migration into the stomach. Clin Imaging. 2021;70:93–6.
5. Lowe AS, Sheridan MB. Esophageal stenting. Semin Intervent Radiol. 2004;21(3):157–66.
6. Hindy P, Hong J, Lam-Tsai Y, Gress F. A comprehensive review of esophageal stents. Gastroenterol Hepatol (NY). 2012;8(8):526–34.
7. Acunas B, Rozanes I, Akpinar S, Tunaci A, Tunaci M, Acunas G. Palliation of malignant esophageal strictures with self-expanding nitinol stents: drawbacks and complications. Radiology. 1996;199:648–52.
8. Baron TH. Expandable metal stents for the treatment of cancerous obstruction of the gastrointestinal tract. N Engl J Med. 2001;344:1681–7.
9. de Gregorio MA, Mainar A, Rodriguez J, Alfonso ER, Tejero E, Herrera M, et al. Colon stenting: a review. Semin Intervent Radiol. 2004;21(3):205–16.
10. Morino M, Arezzo A, Farnesi F, Forcignanò E. Colonic stenting in the emergency setting. Medicina. 2021;57(4):328.
11. Harris G, Senagore A, Lavery I, Fazio V. The management of neoplastic colorectal obstruction with colonic endolumenal stenting devices. Am J Surg. 2001;181:499–506.

Chapter 13
Hepatobiliary and Pancreatic Interventions

Eva Liu and Prasaanthan Gopee-Ramanan

Liver Biopsy

Image-guided biopsy of the liver is undertaken to obtain a tissue sample for pathological diagnosis of a lesion initially identified on imaging. The indication for liver biopsy is used for diagnostic clarification, staging, prognosis, and treatment guidance. An inaccessible lesion, abnormal coagulopathy, or uncooperative patients are all contraindications. The most common type of liver biopsy is percutaneous biopsy where a thin needle is inserted, under ultrasound or computed tomography (CT) guidance, and a small sample of tissue is removed for biopsy.

Patient Preparation

Preparation of the patient consists of:

- Obtaining informed consent, make sure to discuss the option of not having the biopsy.
- Reviewing and correcting (if necessary) coagulation status. Standard transfusion target include hematocrit $\geq 25\%$, platelet count $>50 \times 109/L$, and fibrinogen $>120\,mg/dL$.
- Ensuring fasting for at least 2 h prior.

E. Liu (✉)
Michael G. DeGroote School of Medicine, McMaster University, Hamilton, ON, Canada
e-mail: eva.liu@medportal.ca

P. Gopee-Ramanan
Department of Radiology, Michael G. DeGroote School of Medicine, Faculty of Health Sciences, McMaster University, Hamilton, ON, Canada
e-mail: prasa.gopee@medportal.ca

Complications from liver biopsy include:

- Hemorrhage
- AV fistula formation
- Infection
- Biliary sepsis

Post-procedural care depends on the:

- Nature of the patient's condition
- Location of the biopsy
- Complications encountered
- Coagulation status

Generally, vital signs are monitored every 15 min for 1 h, every 30 min for the next 2 h, and every 2 h after that until deemed ready for discharge. Analgesia may be administered as needed. Most commonly, patients are advised bed rest for 2–3 h, and vital signs are monitored for the same duration.

Percutaneous Biliary Drainage and Stenting

Indications and Contraindications

- Indications for percutaneous biliary drainage and stenting (Fig. 13.1) include obstructive jaundice as a result of malignant or benign biliary stricture or treatment of cholangitis when ERCP or surgery is not possible.
- Ascites is a relative contraindication.

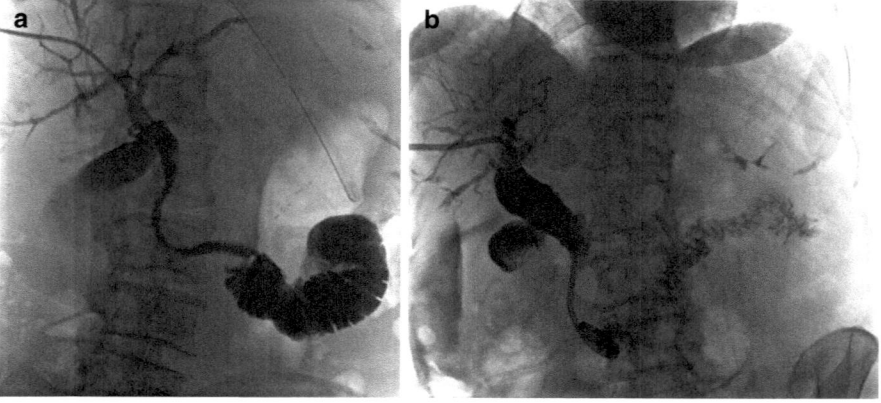

Fig. 13.1 (**a**) Percutaneous transhepatic biliary drainage and stent. (**b**) Percutaneous transhepatic internal\external biliary drainage

Procedure

Prophylactic single dose of antibiotics as per local policy is given. Under fluoroscopy or adjunct ultrasound guidance, local anesthetic is infiltrated into the liver capsule via approaching through the intercostal space above the tenth rib at the midaxillary line. A Chiba (22G) needle is inserted and advanced under fluoroscopy toward the xiphisternum until it reaches the transverse process of the vertebral body. After removing the central stylet, contrast medium is slowly injected while pulling back on the needle until an intrahepatic duct is breached, and a swirling of bile and contrast medium is visualized. Once the ductal location is confirmed, a guide wire is advanced toward the CBD, the Chiba needle is removed, and a Ness set is introduced over the wire. A hydrophilic wire is advanced through the Ness set and is negotiated down the CBD. A larger 6–8 F sheath is then inserted, injecting contrast medium as needed to visualize the stricture. A 5 Fr Kumpe (Cook) catheter might be employed to negotiate the hydrophilic wire down the CBD and also across the stricture. The hydrophilic wire is then exchanged for the Amplatz wire and then the tract is dilated. An internal\external biliary drain or a biliary stent can then be left in place [1].

Complications

Complications include:

- Bleeding
- Biliary peritonitis
- Sepsis [1]

Cholecystostomy Drainage

Percutaneous cholecystostomy decompresses the gallbladder under fluoroscopic guidance and/or ultrasound guidance (Fig. 13.2). This reduces symptoms and inflammation from acute cholecystitis. It is most useful in high-risk patients as a bridging therapy to cholecystectomy [2]. The procedure is very similar to percutaneous biliary drainage and stenting discussed previously. The two options for approach are transhepatic and transperitoneal, as dictated by patient condition and anatomy. In the case of a transhepatic approach, care must be exercised to avoid damage to the lung, pleura, or neurovascular bundle inferior to the rib. For the transperitoneal approach, T-fasteners may be used to further anchor the gallbladder to the wall, especially since it is expected that decompression over time will cause some shifting of the gallbladder and drain. The procedure is ended with a cholecystogram to ensure adequate drainage [2].

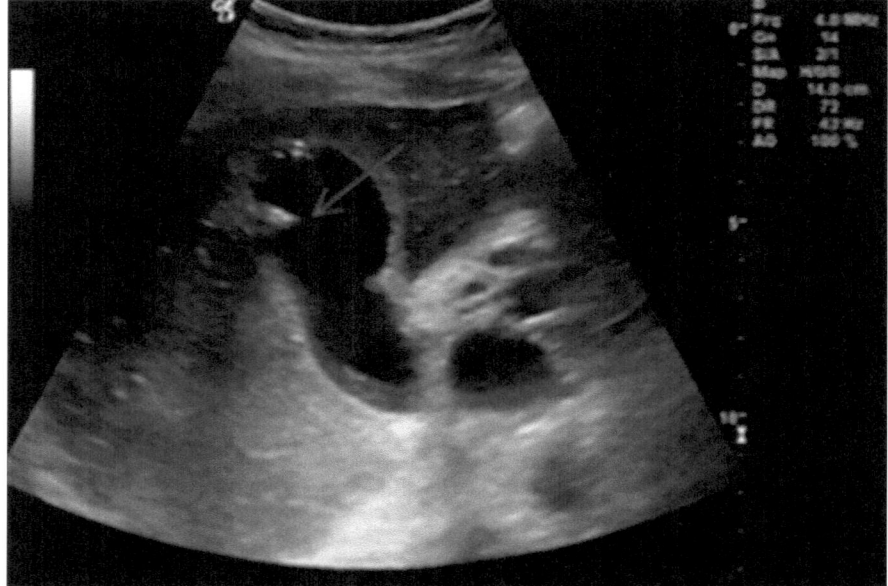

Fig. 13.2 Ultrasound image showing the pigtail cholecystostomy tube (*arrow*) within the gallbladder

Transarterial Chemoembolization

Clinical Background

Hepatocellular carcinoma (HCC) is the most common primary liver malignancy and sixth most common malignancy worldwide. Key risk factors include hepatitis B/C infection (HBV/HCV), alcoholic liver damage, nonalcoholic steatohepatitis (NASH), and exposure to aflatoxin B1. The premise of TACE is to induce ischemia of tumor bed and increase susceptibility or response to chemotherapeutic agents, such as sorafenib.

Diagnosis

The current gold standard for HCC screening includes the HCC biomarker alpha-fetoprotein (AFP) and ultrasonography on the basis of cost-effectiveness [3]. Levels exceeding 400 ng/mL (normal <10 ng/mL) have an HCC positive predictive value of 95% [4]. If suspicious nodules are detected, the American Association for the Study of Liver Diseases (AASLD) recommendations are for liver nodules <1 cm on ultrasonography to be observed ultrasonographically every 3 months until either stability or growth of the lesion is established [5].

Classification

TNM cancer staging is widely used for prognostic purposes in patients who can undergo surgical resection or transplantation [5–7]. The Americas Hepato-Pancreato-Biliary Association/American Joint Committee on Cancer (AHPBA/AJCC) 2010 consensus statement recommends use of the Barcelona Clinic Liver Cancer (BCLC) staging system in patients with advanced liver disease who are not surgical candidates (Fig. 13.3) [8]. Liver Imaging and Reporting Data System (LI-RADS) seeks to standardize imaging reports by radiology for HCC diagnosis and staging [10].

Treatment Options

Current treatments for HCC available in interventional radiology include:

- Transarterial chemoembolization (TACE)
- Radiofrequency ablation (RFA)
- Cryoablation

Treatment decision for HCC is complicated due to the heterogeneity of the disease, overlying liver disorders, and requires input from a multidisciplinary team of hepatologists, interventional radiologists, medical oncologists, and surgical oncologists.

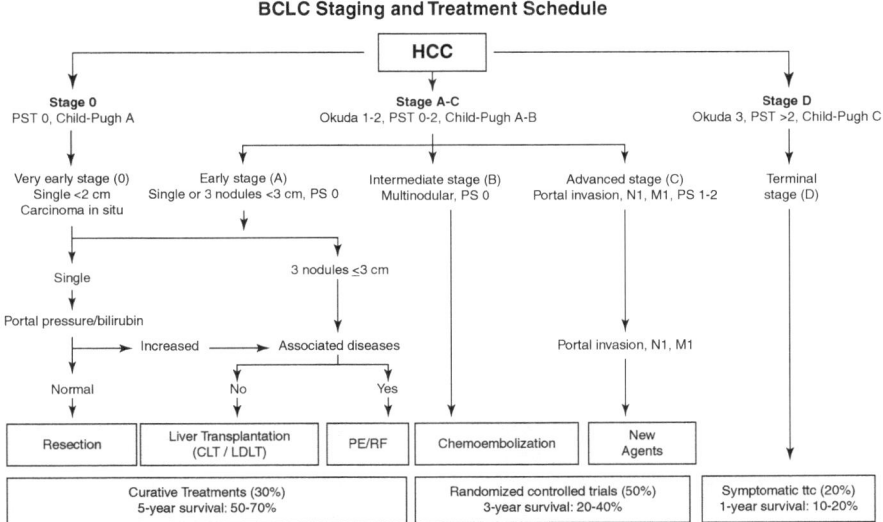

Fig. 13.3 BCLC staging and treatment schedule [8, 9]

TACE

TACE involves injection of a cytotoxic drug such as doxorubicin that has been emulsified radio-opaque agents followed by embolic agents (discussed more in Chap. 9) into selective hepatic artery branches providing blood flow to a tumor [11]. TACE can be used to treat patients who do not meet criteria for resection and to serve as a bridge therapy until transplant; it is the current standard for patients with intermediate stage HCC. Drug-eluting beads (DEB) are embolic microspheres loaded with cytotoxic drugs used to achieve sustained cytotoxicity. However, despite the promise of DEB-TACE, randomized controlled trials have failed to show superiority compared to conventional TACE in terms of patient survival, tumor response, and safety [11]. Recent comparison of TACE-RFA with RFA alone has shown improved survival in patients with HCC tumors less than 7 cm having received TACE-RFA combination therapy [12]. Treatment allocation, tumor size, and tumor number were significant prognostic factors for overall survival, whereas treatment allocation and tumor number were significant prognostic factors for recurrence-free survival [12].

Contraindications

Absolute contraindications include [13, 14]:

- Decompensated cirrhosis (Child-Pugh B or higher) including:

  - Jaundice
  - Clinical encephalopathy
  - Refractory ascites
  - Hepatorenal syndrome

- Extensive tumor with massive replacement of both lobes
- Severely reduced portal vein flow (e.g., non-tumoral portal vein occlusion or hepatofugal blood flow)
- Technical contraindications to hepatic intra-arterial treatment (e.g., untreatable arteriovenous fistula)
- Renal insufficiency (creatinine 2 mg/dL or creatinine clearance 30 mL/min)

  Relative contraindications include [13, 14]:

- Tumor size >10 cm
- Comorbidities involving compromised organ function:

  - Active cardiovascular disease
  - Active lung disease

- Untreated varices at high risk of bleeding
- Bile duct occlusion or incompetent papilla due to stent or surgery

Common Embolic Agents

Temporary agents include Gelfoam, and permanent agents include particles (e.g., PVA), coils, and liquid agents (e.g., glue, onyx).

Treatment Outcomes

TACE is shown to improve median survival by 16–20 months [15], and use of embolic drug-eluting beads (DEB) via TACE has improved the pharmacokinetics of TACE and reduced systemic drug exposure [15]. DEB-TACE combination is currently being investigated [15].

Complications

Complications include:

- Access site injury
- Hepatic artery injury
- Pulmonary embolism

Imaging Required

Pre-procedure:

- Triple-phase computed tomography (CT) or magnetic resonance imaging (MRI) of the liver
- Additional images as needed to rule out extrahepatic disease [15]

Radioembolization

The subdivision of interventional oncology under interventional radiology is seeing a greater implementation of liver-directed therapies for management of unresectable primary and secondary liver tumors, colorectal cancers, and neuroendocrine tumors. Treatment with radioembolization involves administering non-embolic glass or resin microspheres containing radioactive yttrium-90. Under fluoroscopic guidance, once access to the vasculature feeding the tumor is achieved under fluoroscopic guidance, the microspheres are slowly injected with intermittent contrast medium and sterile water [16]. Although there are no randomized control trials at this time comparing radioembolization to transarterial chemoembolization (TACE) or its drug-eluting bead variant, comparative literature shows reduced toxicity and a trend toward greater survival benefit with radioembolization [17]. Radioembolization is also more suitable for patients with multiple lesions. Further work is being carried out to look for radiofrequency ablation prior to or following radioembolization [16].

There have been more recent updated trials surrounding Y-90 and hepatocellular carcinoma which are worth citing here. Woerner and Johnson (2022) [18] published a paper surrounding the role of this form of radioembolization therapy with treatment goals and considerations for different stages of disease.

Fiorentini et al. (2020) [19] have also recently published an update on the use of DEBIRI therapy in the management of disseminated colorectal cancer which are otherwise not responsive to chemo- or immunotherapy and not surgically resectable.

Acknowledgment We would like to thank Dr. Prasaanthan Gopee-Ramanan for his contributions to this chapter (information given on first page of chapter).

References

1. Krokidis M, Orgera G, Rossi M, et al. Interventional radiology in the management of benign biliary stenoses, biliary leaks and fistulas: a pictorial review. Insights Imaging. 2013;4(1):77–84.
2. Little MW, Briggs JH, Tapping CR, et al. Percutaneous cholecystostomy: the radiologist's role in treating acute cholecystitis. Clin Radiol. 2013;68(7):654–60.
3. Thompson Coon J, Rogers G, Hewson P, et al. Surveillance of cirrhosis for hepatocellular carcinoma: systematic review and economic analysis. Health Technol Assess. 2007;11(34):1–206.
4. Singal AG, Conjeevaram HS, Volk ML, et al. Effectiveness of hepatocellular carcinoma surveillance in patients with cirrhosis. Cancer Epidemiol Biomark Prev. 2012;21(5):793–9.
5. Bruix J, Sherman M. American association for the study of liver diseases. Management of hepatocellular carcinoma: an update. Hepatology. 2011;53(3):1020–2.
6. Vauthey JN, Dixon E, Abdalla EK, et al. Pretreatment assessment of hepatocellular carcinoma: expert consensus statement. HPB (Oxford). 2010;12(5):289–99.
7. Kadri HS, Blank S, Wang Q, et al. Outcomes following liver resection and clinical pathologic characteristics of hepatocellular carcinoma occurring in patients with chronic hepatitis B and minimally fibrotic liver. Eur J Surg Oncol. 2013;39(12):1371–6.
8. Llovet JM, Burroughs A, Bruix J. Hepatocellular carcinoma. Lancet. 2003;362:1907–17.
9. Kennedy SA, Gopee-Ramanan P, Dath D. Hepatocellular carcinoma: a clinical review. MUMJ. 2014;11(1):9–14.
10. Tang A, Cruite I, Sirlin CB. Toward a standardized system for hepatocellular carcinoma diagnosis using computed tomography and MRI. Expert Rev Gastroenterol Hepatol. 2013;7(3):269–79.
11. Raoul JL, Forner A, Bolondi L, Cheung TT, Kloeckner R, de Baere T. Updated use of TACE for hepatocellular carcinoma treatment: how and when to use it based on clinical evidence. Cancer Treat Rev. 2019;72:28–36.
12. Peng ZW, Zhang YJ, Chen MS, et al. Radiofrequency ablation with or without transcatheter arterial chemoembolization in the treatment of hepatocellular carcinoma: a prospective randomized trial. J Clin Oncol. 2013;31(4):426–32.
13. Lencioni R, Petruzzi P, Crocetti L. Chemoembolization of hepatocellular carcinoma. Semin Intervent Radiol. 2013;30(1):3–11.

14. Raoul JL, Sangro B, Forner A, et al. Evolving strategies for the management of intermediate-stage hepatocellular carcinoma: available evidence and expert opinion on the use of transarterial chemoembolization. Cancer Treat Rev. 2011;37(3):212–20.
15. Steward MJ, Warbey VS, Malhotra A, et al. Neuroendocrine tumors: role of interventional radiology in therapy. Radiographics. 2008;28(4):1131–45.
16. Bester L, Meteling B, Boshell D, et al. Transarterial chemoembolisation and radioembolisation for the treatment of primary liver cancer and secondary liver cancer: a review of the literature. J Med Imaging Radiat Oncol. 2014;58(3):341–52.
17. Salem R, Lewandowski R, Atassi B. Treatment of unresectable hepatocellular carcinoma with use of Y90 microspheres (TheraSphere): safety, tumor response, and survival. J Vasc Interv Radiol. 2005;16:1627–39.
18. Woerner AJ, Johnson GE. Advances in Y-90 radioembolization for the treatment of hepatocellular carcinoma. Hepatoma Res. 2022;8:2.
19. Fiorentini G, Sarti D, Nani R, Aliberti C, Fiorentini C, Guadagni S. Updates of colorectal cancer liver metastases therapy: review on DEBIRI. Hepat Oncol. 2020;7(1):HEP16.

Chapter 14
Genitourinary Interventions

**Ibrahim Mohammad Nadeem, Ruqqiyah Rana,
and Prasaanthan Gopee-Ramanan**

Kidney Biopsy

Percutaneous image-guided renal biopsy is the gold standard for the diagnosis of renal parenchymal diseases. The procedure allows for accurate and reliable method of acquiring renal tissue for histopathological assessment. Biopsy can be performed under CT or ultrasound. Choice of modality depends on both patient and operator factors. Alternative for percutaneous image-guided renal biopsy is transjugular renal biopsy.

Indications and Contraindications

Indications for renal biopsy include:

- Renal failure without a clinically evident cause
- Nephrotic syndrome

I. M. Nadeem (✉) · P. Gopee-Ramanan
Department of Radiology, Faculty of Health Sciences, McMaster University,
Hamilton, ON, Canada
e-mail: ibrahim.nadeem@medportal.ca; prasa.gopee@medportal.ca

R. Rana
Michael G. DeGroote School of Medicine, McMaster University, Hamilton, ON, Canada
e-mail: ruqqiyah.rana@medportal.ca

S. Athreya, M. Albahhar (eds.), *Demystifying Interventional Radiology*,
https://doi.org/10.1007/978-3-031-12023-7_14

135

- Glomerular nephritis
- Focal lesions non-characterized on diagnostic imaging
- Renal transplant rejection

  Contraindications include:

- Uncorrected coagulopathy.
- Atrophic.
- Scarred kidneys.
- Heavy burden of polycystic kidney disease.
- Relatively bleeding diathesis.
- Uncontrolled hypertension.
- Pyelonephritis.
- Morbid obesity.
- Ascites.
- Other general contraindications for any biopsy also apply.

Patient Preparation

Preparation of the patient consists of:

- Obtaining informed consent
- Reviewing and correcting (if necessary) coagulation status
- Ensuring fasting for at least 2 h prior

Procedure

The patient is positioned prone, and the procedure is usually guided by ultrasound and occasionally by CT. The target area for specimen retrieval is identified to either the upper or lower pole of the kidney. Local anesthetic is injected from the skin to the renal capsule. Usually an 18-G core biopsy needle under ultrasound guidance is advanced into the kidney, and 2–3 biopsies are taken. Direct pressure is then applied to the needle entry site for several minutes followed by monitoring of blood pressure.

A similar procedure is target lesion kidney biopsy which is performed mainly for further evaluation and diagnosis of renal tumors. Targeted biopsies are distinct from non-targeted biopsies in that they are performed with the intention of specifically identifying the nature of a discrete lesion or lesions, as identified on imaging; non-targeted biopsies extract tissue from anywhere within the renal parenchyma to diagnose renal diseases which affect the kidney more diffusely.

Complications

- Hemorrhage is the most common complication, and in kidney biopsies, this manifests as hematuria for up to 24 h.
- Severe bleeding requiring aggressive measures, including nephrectomy, may occur in less than 1% of cases.
- Other complications include infection, AV fistula formation, pneumothorax, or injury to nearby viscera.

Post-procedural Care

Post-procedural care depends on the:

- Nature of the patient's condition
- Location of the biopsy
- Complications encountered
- Coagulation status

Generally, vital signs are monitored every 15 min for 1 h, every 30 min for the next 2 h, and every 2 h after that until deemed ready to discontinue. Analgesia may be administered as needed.

Transjugular Renal Biopsy

Transjugular renal biopsy is usually performed in settings where percutaneous renal biopsy is not feasible or contraindicated. At present, only a few centers perform this procedure.

Indications

The most frequent indications for performing transjugular instead of percutaneous biopsy are [1]:

- Infracostal kidneys
- Morbid obesity
- COPD with postural disability
- Retroperitoneal tumor mass

- Uncorrected coagulopathy
- Thrombocytopenia
- Patients with single kidney
- Other unspecified percutaneous puncture difficulties/impossibilities

Procedure [1]

The following steps should be followed:

- With the patient in supine position, patency of the internal jugular veins is assessed using ultrasound.
- Under ultrasound guidance, the right internal jugular vein is punctured with an 18-guage needle, and a 7- or 9-F venous sheath is inserted.
- Under fluoroscopic control and with a multipurpose catheter and hydrophilic guide, the catheter is advanced into the inferior vena cava, and the right renal vein is catheterized. The transjugular renal biopsy needle is filled with normal saline and advanced down the catheter.
- All biopsies are performed using the transjugular renal biopsy set. An average of three cores per patient is obtained. The sample is evaluated by a nephrologist at the time of extraction to ensure an adequate number of intact glomeruli were extracted to make a pathological diagnosis.
- The apparatus is removed, and direct pressure is applied to the needle entry site for several minutes followed by monitoring of blood pressure.

Post-procedural Care

All patients are returned to the ward for routine 24-h bed rest and hemodynamic observation. Generally, vitals are monitored every 15 min for the first 2 h, every 30 min for the next 4 h, and then hourly. Follow-up ultrasound is done 3 h after procedure and on post-procedure day 3.

Complications [1]

- Pain
- Microscopic hematuria
- Peripuncture jugular bleeding
- Asymptomatic perirenal hematoma
- Fornix rupture requiring transfusion

Percutaneous Nephrostomy Drainage

In acute obstructive uropathy, several etiologies can lead to impairment of antegrade peristalsis of the ureters enabling draining of urine from the kidneys to the bladder. Urine stagnation increases risk of urosepsis. Percutaneous nephrostomy drains are useful as an emergent measure for decompression of obstructed urinary collecting systems. Ultrasound-guided introduction of a sheathed needle is done into the most dilated calyx (generally mid-lower pole calyx), with confirmation using contrast media and fluoroscopy. Aspirated urine is sent for culture and sensitivity. Following serial dilatation, a pigtail catheter is inserted into the renal pelvis and secured, and a drainage bag is attached. Mortality rate from complications is low at 0.046–0.3% [2].

Clinical Background

Antegrade peristalsis of the ureters allows physiological drainage of the kidneys to the bladder. Radiation changes, surgery, inflammation, and malignancy can compress and impede this drainage by resulting in acute obstructive uropathy [3], and stagnant urine in the collecting system can predispose to sepsis. Percutaneous nephrostomy as treatment of hydronephrosis dates back to 1955 and is particularly useful as an emergent measure for decompression of obstructed urinary collecting systems [4].

Indications and Contraindications

Indications include:

- Acute obstructive uropathy

  Contraindications include:

- Hemodynamic instability
- Unmanaged coagulopathy

Pre-procedure

- Chart review and coagulation screen are performed and informed consent obtained.
- In addition, INR <1.5 and platelet count >50,000/mm^3 [5] are ensured, and patients with allergies to contrast media should be premeditated as per departmental protocol.

- Ensure hemodynamic stability, which is achieved by intravenous fluids, antibiotics, and vasopressors [6].
- Anesthesiology may be involved in severely septic patients to ensure hemodynamic stability.
- Ensure the patient is NPO, and review previous imaging (ultrasound, computed tomography, etc.) to plan the procedure and anticipate complications and avoid damage to nearby organs.

Procedure

The patient is positioned prone on a fluoroscopy table with the procedure side closest to the interventional radiologist. A small pillow or positioning wedge should be placed to angle the patient 20–30° toward the interventional radiologist allowing for needle trajectory along the avascular plane of Brodel [5, 7]. Following ultrasound evaluation of the position, a wide area from the lower thorax to the iliac crest is prepared with chlorhexidine solution and draped. Local anesthesia is given using 10 mL of 1% lidocaine.

Ultrasound-guided introduction of a sheathed needle (Chiba needle) is done into the most dilated calyx, ideally below the 12th rib to avoid complications such as pneumothorax or empyema [7]. Confirming needle placement in the calyx, the inner stylet is removed, and urine is aspirated into a syringe to send off for culture and sensitivity (if urosepsis is known).

Following the initial decompression of the collecting system, a 1:1 diluted water-soluble contrast medium is injected into the renal pelvis under fluoroscopy. Following the insertion of a guide wire into the collecting system, the needle is removed, and the Ness set is introduced over the wire. The tract is serially dilated using 6-F and 8-F dilators for 8-F drainage catheters; 10-F or 12-F dilators may be considered for 10–12-F drainage catheters when there is thick pus [5, 7]. Pigtail tip positioning of the catheter is confirmed via contrast administration under fluoroscopy. The catheter is then secured and a drainage bag attached.

Post-procedure

- Following the procedure, monitor vital signs and maintain the patient on antibiotics as appropriate.
- During post-procedure days 1 and 2, monitor vitals, WBC, nephrostomy tube output volume, and urinary output, and check culture results. Tube patency can be maintained via flushing using 10 mL of normal saline.
- Hemorrhage and hematoma within the collecting system do not require any special management of the tube [7]. If significant hemorrhagic output is noted, then catheter injection with contrast medium can be performed to assess for renal vasculature involvement or pseudoaneurysm formation.

Complications

Mortality rates from complications are low at 0.046–0.3% [2].

- Hematuria is transiently expected and will resolve in 48–72 h. Larger clots in the collecting system may be broken down by urokinase in urine, but hematocrit vital signs should be monitored in the days following the procedure.
- Untreated bacterial sepsis upon decompression of the vascular bed can occur in 2.5% of cases, even occurring ten times more in patients with pyelonephritis [7]. Sepsis post-procedure is avoided by administering antibiotic prophylaxis, decompression of the collecting system prior to contrast medium injection, slow injection of contrast medium, and selective or minimal manipulation of guide wires; careful post-procedural monitoring is key.
- Other complications that may occur are injury to the liver, spleen, pleura, or colon during needle insertion.

Ureteral Stenting

Antegrade percutaneous internal/external nephroureteral (PCNU) stents allow both internal and external drainage of urine from the renal pelvis (Figs. 14.1 and 14.2). Externally, the drain segment can be connected to gravity drainage if there is an obstruction preventing internal drainage of urine to the bladder. Otherwise, this external segment can be capped but left in place, thereby allowing internal filling of the ureter and urinary bladder but leaving in place an option for flushing of the stent or reversion to external gravity drainage, if needed [8]. Indications for PCNU placement include benign or malignant obstructions, in conjunction with extracorporeal shock wave lithotripsy (ESWL), and maintenance of ureteral patency while allowing for postoperative healing (thereby preventing stricture formation) [9].

Procedure

The procedure begins with a nephrostogram. Depending on the pathology, a decision can be made to initially place a percutaneous nephrostomy allowing for decompression. This can then be converted to a PCNU.

Under conscious sedation and following administration of a single dose of antibiotics, the patient is positioned prone, and access to the kidney is gained via the avascular plane of Brodel as for percutaneous nephrostomy. A standard guide wire is inserted anterograde into the renal pelvis and then the ureter, and a catheter is passed over it. A water-soluble contrast can be used with fluoroscopy to confirm. Then the guide wire is exchanged for a hydrophilic one and the obstruction is negotiated. Confirming with contrast that the distal catheter tip has reached past the

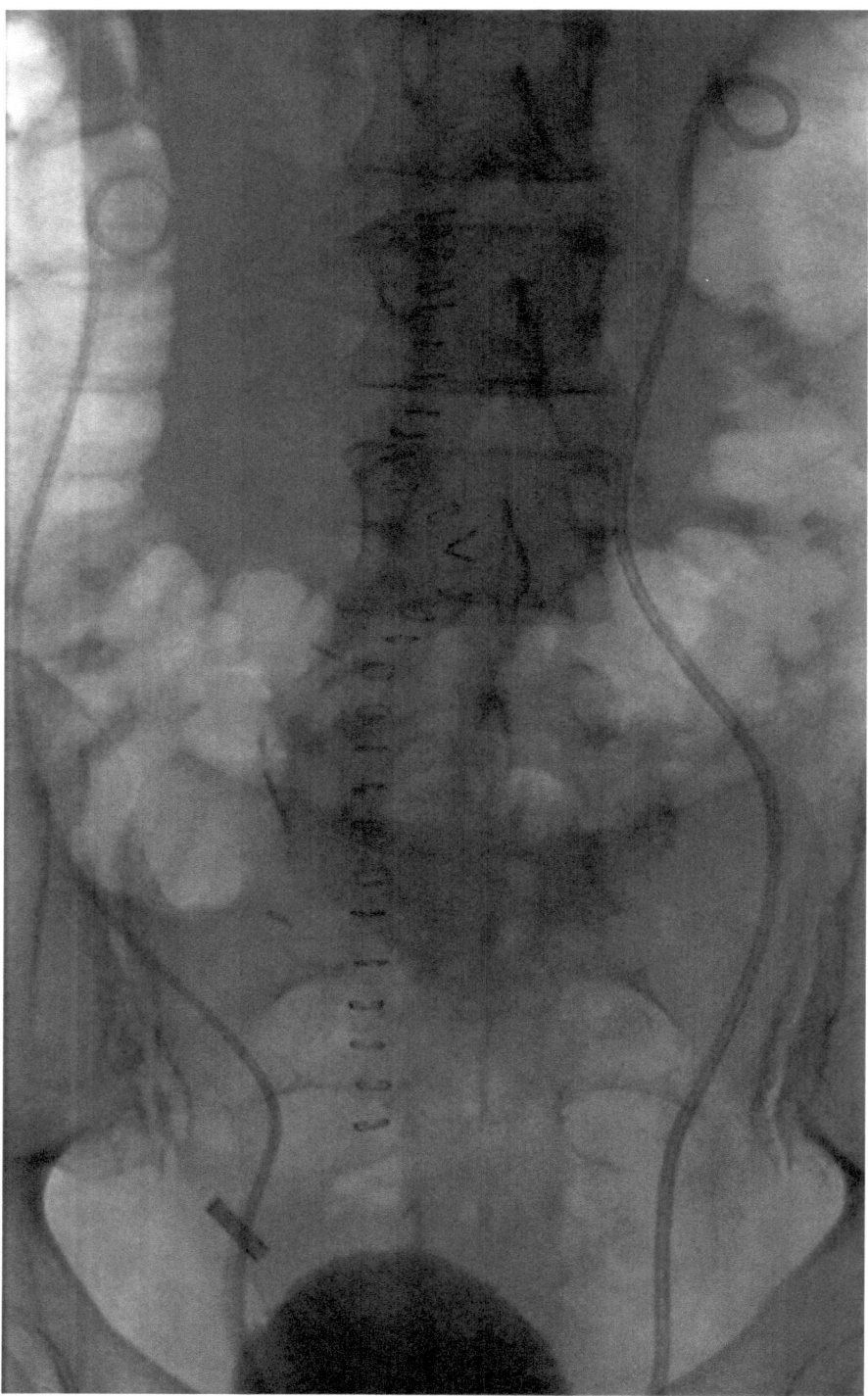

Fig. 14.1 Bilateral ureteral stents

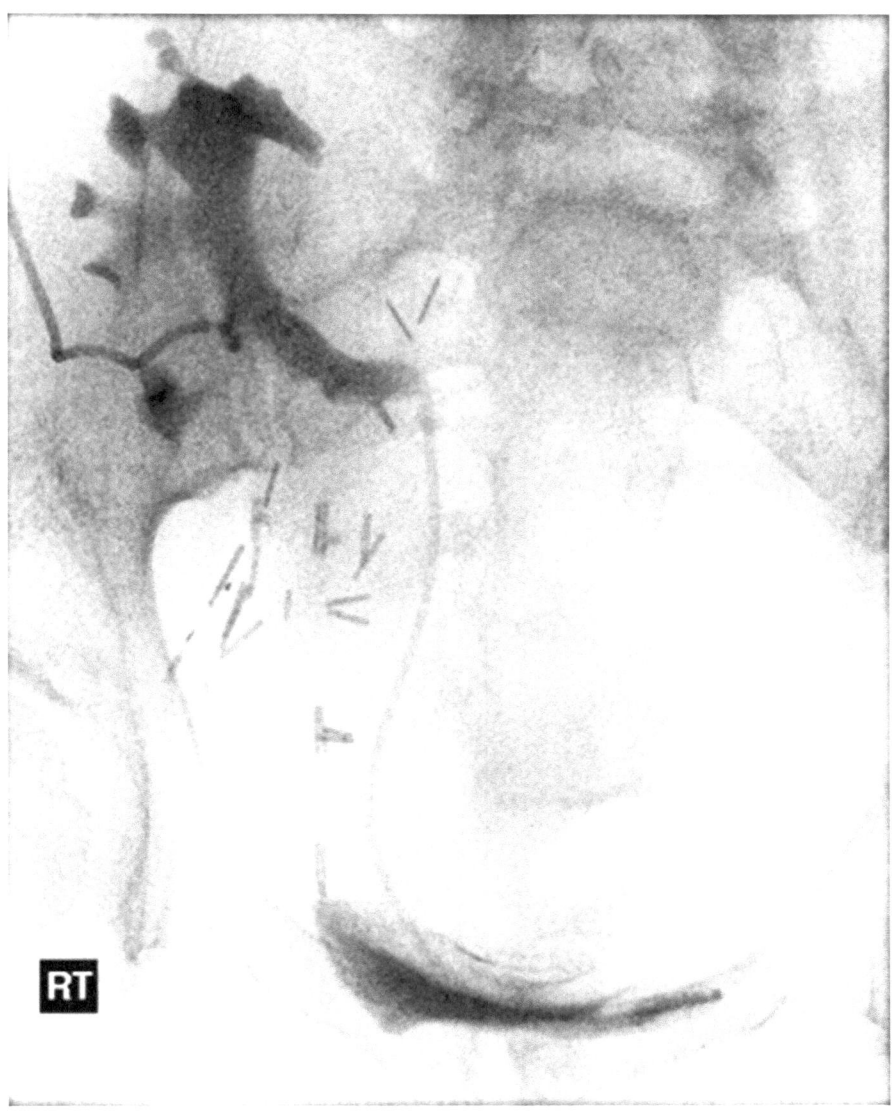

Fig. 14.2 Renal transplant nephroureterostomy

ureterovesicular junction (UVJ), the hydrophilic guide wire is again replaced with the stiff one, and the stent system is deployed. A balloon dilator may be used in the case of a difficult obstruction. Once the stent is in place, adequate drainage is confirmed via contrast injection under fluoroscopy. If there is bleeding noted and a clot has formed in the drainage system during the procedure, a nephrostomy tube may need to be left in place for 24–48 h.

Complications

Common complications include:

- Irritative bladder symptoms
- Loin pain
- Infections
- Hematuria
- Migration, or decreased efficacy

  Uncommon complications include:

- Stent fracture or ureteral erosion [8, 9]

Suprapubic Catheter Insertion

Suprapubic catheterization, also referred to as suprapubic cystostomy, is indicated whenever there is urinary obstruction, but a transurethral catheter is contraindicated (e.g., urethral disruption) or technically unfeasible. The bladder should be distended for safe access (an undistended bladder has the risk of transperitoneal access and bowel injury).

Procedure

- The patient is positioned supine. Following local anesthetic infiltration, a 20-G spinal needle is advanced suprapubically.
- An 18- or 19-G sheath needle is inserted under ultrasound guidance, and a super-stiff catheter is passed intraluminally into the bladder.
- Once enough guide wire is curled within the urinary bladder, serial dilation of the tract is carried out.
- A peel-away sheath 2 F larger than the final Foley or pigtail drainage catheter to be used is then inserted into the tract.
- Once the Foley or pigtail drainage catheter is inserted, the balloon is distended with 7–10 mL of sterile water, and the peel-away sheath is removed.

Complications

Complications include:

- Hematuria

- Skin infections
- Bowel perforations or visceral organ damage
- Recurrent urinary tract infections

Renal Artery Angioplasty and Stenting

Renal artery stenosis (RAS) is the most common cause of secondary hypertension, with over 90% of cases being caused by atherosclerosis and the rest mainly by fibromuscular dysplasia (FMD) [10]. Percutaneous angioplasty and stenting are an option for management of renal artery stenosis, with excellent results shown to reduce systemic hypertension and preserve renal function (Figs. 14.3 and 14.4). The location of this disease renders it less well treated by balloon angioplasty alone; thus, balloon expandable stenting is preferred [11].

Contraindications include:

- Branch vessel disease
- Kidney size smaller than 7 cm
- Uncooperative patients
- Stenoses longer than 2 cm
- Intrarenal vascular disease [11]

Generally, technical success rates are 80–99% [12]. Complications include:

- Renal artery dissection
- Transection
- Thrombosis
- Embolization [11]

Although small retrospective studies have shown some modest benefit of renal artery angioplasty and stenting for patients, there is a lack of strong evidence supporting revascularization of RAS versus medical management based on published randomized control trials thus far [13, 14].

The Cardiovascular Outcomes in Renal Atherosclerotic Lesions (CORAL) trial is the most recent to investigate the role for endovascular versus medical management for RAS: it essentially concluded that renal artery stenting in people with RAS offers no advantages over best medical therapy in reducing hard clinical events. This is in keeping with American College of Cardiology and American Heart Association guidelines recommending renal artery stenting as a reasonable option for patients with one of the following: an atherosclerotic severe renal artery stenosis (greater than 70% angiographic diameter renal artery stenosis or 50–70% stenosis with hemodynamic confirmation of lesion severity) associated with (1) resistant or uncontrolled hypertension and the failure of three antihypertensive drugs, one of which is a diuretic agent, and (2) hypertension and intolerance to medication [15, 16].

Fig. 14.3 (**a**) CT angiogram showing left renal artery stenosis. (**b**) Angiogram showing bilateral renal artery stenosis

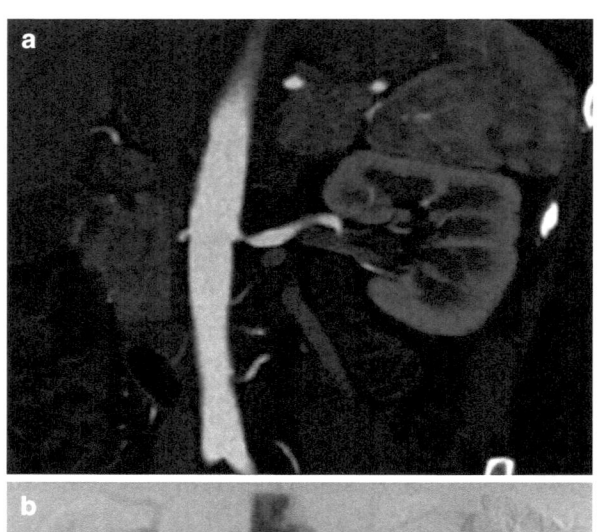

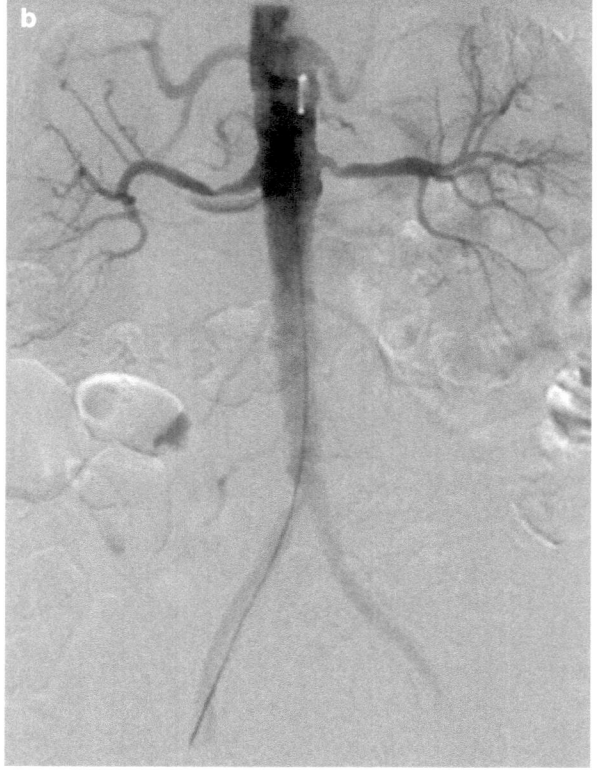

Fig. 14.4 (**a**) Post-angioplasty and stenting of left renal artery stenosis. (**b**) Angiogram showing stented right renal artery stenosis

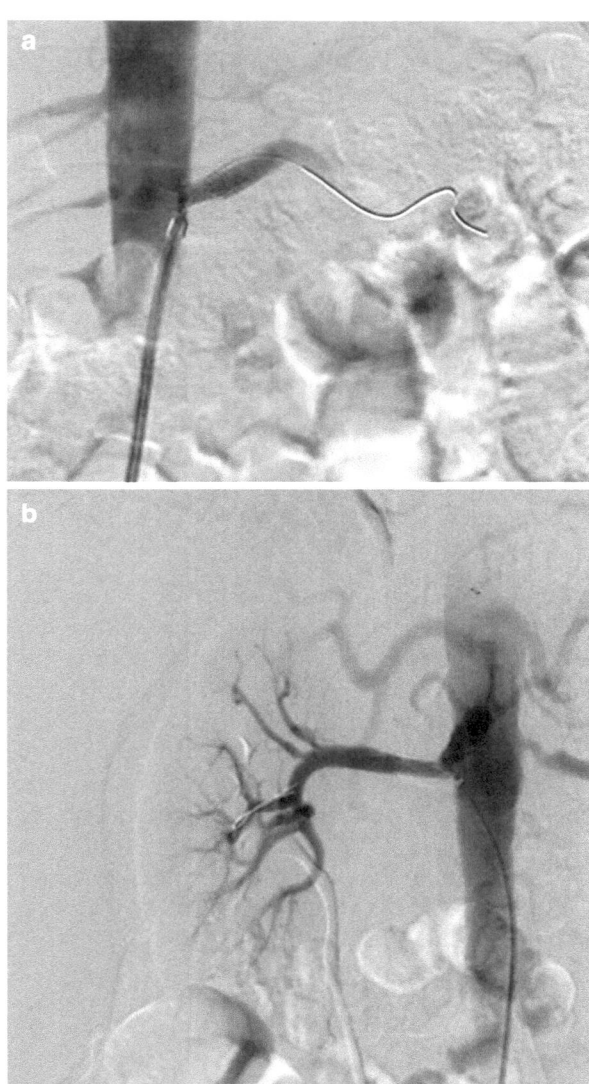

Prostatic Artery Embolization

Prostatic artery embolization (PAE) for benign prostatic hypertrophy (BPH) as a primary alternative to the "gold standard" of transurethral resection of the prostate (TURP) is beginning to show promise [17–19]. Selection of patients and technical proficiency are seen to be key in outcome analysis [17]. Due to the complexity of prostatic vascular anatomy and the burden from atherosclerosis, thin arteries, and comorbidities in elderly patients, experienced interventional radiologists must carry out the procedure preferably [17]. A single dose of ciprofloxacin is administered prior to the procedure followed by a 7-day course of the same.

- A Foley balloon containing a mixture of iodinate contrast medium and normal saline allows for better visualization of the prostate and surrounding vessels to avoid collateral procedural damage.
- The key arteries feeding the prostate are first localized by angiography. Generally, the inferior vesicular artery is catheterized using the road map technique with contrast medium under fluoroscopy.
- The embolic agents of choice are then mixed with normal saline and iodinate contrast media and injected at a slow rate under fluoroscopy.
- Embolization may take 10–15 min. Depending on the nature of the anatomy encountered, a follow-up angiogram may be warranted once stasis is confirmed to look for any collateral supply. Generally, there are no significant side effects.
- Clinical success is reflected on the improvement of lower urinary tract symptoms over time [17–19].

Evidence also supports offering PAE to prostate cancer patients symptomatic of bleeding earlier on in their management, prior to palliative radiation therapy in patients with advanced disease. Further research has been carried out to elucidate the role of placebo versus true benefit from PAE for BPH and establishment of safety and effectiveness studies prior to a randomized control study. New and emerging research conducted as recently as of February 2022 have vouched for its efficacy and safety and have shown benefit in patients wishing to avoid surgical procedures or those contraindicated for surgical procedures [20].

Acknowledgment We would like to thank Prasaanthan Gopee-Ramanan for his contributions to this chapter (information given on first page of chapter).

References

1. Bolufer M, García-Carro C, Agraz I, et al. Utility of transjugular renal biopsy as an alternative to percutaneous biopsy. Biopsia renal transyugular. La alternativa a la biopsia percutánea en pacientes de alto riesgo. Nefrologia (Engl Ed). 2020;40(6):634–9. https://doi.org/10.1016/j.nefro.2020.04.018.
2. Ferral H, Stackhouse DJ, Bjarnason H, et al. Complications of percutaneous nephrostomy tube placement. Semin Intervent Radiol. 1994;11:198–206.
3. Adamo R, Saad WE, Brown DB. Percutaneous ureteral interventions. Tech Vasc Interv Radiol. 2009;12(3):205–15.
4. Goodwin WE, Casey WC, Woolf W. Percutaneous trocar (needle) nephrostomy in hydronephrosis. JAMA. 1955;157:891–4.
5. Dyer RB, Regan JD, Kavanagh PV, et al. Percutaneous nephrostomy with extensions of the technique: step by step. Radiographics. 2002;22:503–25.

6. McDermott VG, Schuster MG, Smith TP. Antibiotic prophylaxis in vascular and interventional radiology. Am J Roentgenol. 1997;169:31–8.
7. Uppot RN. Emergent nephrostomy tube placement for acute urinary obstruction. Tech Vasc Interv Radiol. 2009;12(2):154–61.
8. Makramalla A, Zuckerman DA. Nephroureteral stents: principles and techniques. Semin Intervent Radiol. 2011;28(4):367–79.
9. Lang E. Antegrade ureteral stenting for dehiscence, strictures, and fistulae. AJR Am J Roentgenol. 1984;143(4):795–801.
10. Safian RD, Textor SC. Renal-artery stenosis. N Engl J Med. 2001;314:431–42.
11. Marshall RH, Schiffman MH, Winokur RS, et al. Interventional radiologic techniques for screening, diagnosis and treatment of patients with renal artery stenosis. Curr Urol Rep. 2014;15(6):414.
12. Rees CR. Stents for atherosclerotic renovascular disease. J Vasc Interv Radiol. 1999;10(6):689–705.
13. Wheatley K, Ives N, Gray R, Kalra PA, Moss JG, Baigent C, Carr S, Chalmers N, Eadington D, Hamilton G, Lipkin G, Nicholson A, Scoble J. Revascularization versus medical therapy for renal-artery stenosis. N Engl J Med. 2009;361:1953–62.
14. Sattur S, Prasad H, Bedi U, et al. Renal artery stenosis—an update. Postgrad Med. 2013;125(5):43–50.
15. Hirsch AT, Haskal ZJ, Hertzer NR, et al. ACC/AHA 2005 guidelines for the management of patients with peripheral arterial disease (lower extremity, renal, mesenteric, and abdominal aortic): executive summary a collaborative report from the American Association for Vascular Surgery/Society for Vascular Surgery, Society for Cardiovascular Angiography and Interventions, Society for Vascular Medicine and Biology, Society of Interventional Radiology, and the ACC/AHA Task Force on Practice Guidelines (Writing Committee to Develop Guidelines for the Management of Patients With Peripheral Arterial Disease) endorsed by the American Association of Cardiovascular and Pulmonary Rehabilitation; National Heart, Lung, and Blood Institute; Society for Vascular Nursing; TransAtlantic Inter-Society Consensus; and Vascular Disease Foundation. J Am Coll Cardiol. 2006;47:1239–312.
16. Cooper CJ, Murphy TP, Cutlip DE, et al. Stenting and medical therapy for atherosclerotic renal artery disease. N Engl J Med. 2013; https://doi.org/10.1056/NEJMoa1210753.
17. Carnevale FC, Antunes AA. Prostatic artery embolization for enlarged prostates due to benign prostatic hyperplasia. How I do it. Cardiovasc Intervent Radiol. 2013;36(6):1452–63.
18. Bagla S, Martin CP, Van Breda A, et al. Early results from a United States trial of prostatic artery embolization in the treatment of benign prostatic hyperplasia. J Vasc Interv Radiol. 2014;25(1):47–52.
19. Golzarian J, Antunes AA, Bilhim T, et al. Prostatic artery embolization to treat lower urinary tract symptoms related to benign prostatic hyperplasia and bleeding in patients with prostate cancer: proceedings from a multidisciplinary research consensus panel. J Vasc Interv Radiol. 2014;25(5):665–74.
20. Ibrahim WH, Abduljawad H, Mohamed H, Jamsheer N, Elnaggar ME. Prostatic artery embolization for the treatment of benign prostate hyperplasia: initial experience from Bahrain. Cureus. 2022;14(2):e22593.

Chapter 15
Dialysis Access

Ruqqiyah Rana and Lazar Milovanovic

Background

The selection of hemodialysis access method to be used in a particular patient is dependent on many factors, including

- Indication for dialysis.
- Urgency of dialysis treatment.
- Previous medical conditions and clinical context of the patient.
- Thorough clinical assessment.

Assessment of dialysis access dysfunction should be done on a regular basis through clinical examination and ultrasound, as well as functionality during dialysis procedures. Reduced flow rates or signs of dysfunction should be referred to IR for fistulograms to characterize the dialysis access.

Frequent complications of hemodialysis access may include failure to mature (AVF), venous stenosis, infections, and stent, graft, or vascular thrombosis. There are many percutaneous interventions for dialysis access repair including balloon angioplasty, pharmacologic thrombolysis, and mechanical thrombectomy.

Important Definitions

There are several important definitions utilized by health-care professionals in order to effectively characterize dialysis access patency, complications, and interventions.

R. Rana (✉) · L. Milovanovic
Michael G. DeGroote School of Medicine, McMaster University, Hamilton, ON, Canada
e-mail: ruqqiyah.rana@medportal.ca; lazar.milovanovic@medportal.ca

S. Athreya, M. Albahhar (eds.), *Demystifying Interventional Radiology*,
https://doi.org/10.1007/978-3-031-12023-7_15

These definitions are based on the 2003 SIR guidelines for percutaneous management of dysfunctional dialysis access [1]:

- Thrombosed dialysis access: an AVF or AVG occluded by a thrombus preventing blood flow, diagnosed primarily by physical exam and ultrasound examination.
- Dysfunctional dialysis access: (1) an AVF or AVG with functionally significant stenosis, (2) a native fistula that has not matured within the time period expected, or (3) a dialysis access that cannot be accessed in order to successfully initiate and complete dialysis.
- Functionally significant stenosis: a decrease of more than 50% in vessel diameter of the anastomosed venous drainage system or the graft in addition to abnormalities on hemodynamic or clinical assessment.
- Percutaneous management of thrombosed/dysfunctional dialysis access: an intervention using endovascular techniques in order to maintain or repair dialysis access and ensure sufficient blood flow for dialysis to continue.
- Percutaneous thrombus removal: a procedure to remove a thrombus within the inflow arteries, graft, or outflow veins; may involve pharmacologic thrombolysis and suction, balloon angioplasty, or mechanical thrombectomy.
- Percutaneous treatment of stenosis: a procedure in which normal luminal diameter is restored leading to recovered function of the dialysis access.
- Anatomic success of treated stenosis: an improvement in luminal diameter such that the remaining stenosis is less than or equal to 30% of the original diameter.
- Clinical success of treated stenosis or thrombosis: the ability to resume normal dialysis for at least one session, characterized by the presence of a continuous palpable thrill without pulsation at the area of the arterial anastomosis.
- Hemodynamic success: an improvement and recovery of hemodynamic parameters from reduced values during dialysis access dysfunction.
- Procedural success: an anatomical success along with clinical success or improvement in one or more hemodynamic/clinical indicators.

Arteriovenous Fistula

Overview

Arteriovenous fistulas (AVF) for dialysis access are artificially created connections between arteries and veins without corresponding capillary beds. The first report of surgical AVF creation for dialysis access was published by Brescia and Cimino et al. [2]. Endovascular arteriovenous fistula (endoAVF) is a relatively new minimally-invasive technique of AVF creation. It involves endovascular creation of a side-to-side anastomosis between an adjacent artery and vein, utilizing radiofrequency or thermal energy [3]. There are many different possible locations for AVF creation including the forearm, upper arm, and thigh. Unlike catheters and AVG, AVF do not use any artificial material, reducing risk of infection.

AV Fistula Maturation

Once the fistula is created, it must mature prior to being used for dialysis. Maturation is the process where the high rate of blood flow from the artery through the vein causes dilation and wall thickening of the vein, creating a location for dialysis needle insertion where blood can be removed from and returned to the body at a rapid rate.

Evaluation of AVF maturation is typically done via ultrasound examination, as this modality is largely considered to be most accurate and predictive of AVF maturation [4]. Principle measurements include venous diameter and blood flow rate, although the full list of criteria is given below.

AVF maturation usually takes 6–8 weeks, but may take up to 6 months or even a year in patients, and depends on multiple factors including anatomical location, vessel quality, and collateral flow as well as patient factors including female gender, diabetes, and peripheral vascular disease. The preferred waiting period is 3–4 months after fistula formation [1]. The criteria for adequate AVF dialysis access based on the National Kidney Foundation Kidney Disease Outcomes Quality Initiative (NKF KDOQI) guidelines are presented in Table 15.1 [5].

AVF Locations

- Forearm fistulas can be created by connecting radial artery and cephalic vein.
- Alternative forearm AVF can include brachial artery-cephalic vein fistula and brachial artery-basilic vein fistula.
- Lower extremity: femoral artery-saphenous vein fistula.

Table 15.1 Criteria for adequate AV fistula maturation for dialysis access based on the National Kidney Foundation Kidney Disease Outcomes Quality Initiative (NKF KDOQI) guidelines [5]

Criteria for adequate AVF
AVF reside within 0.6 cm of skin surface
AVF has flow of >600 mL/min
AVF has diameter of >0.6 cm
Maturation in less than 6 weeks

Graft Implantation

Overview

Arteriovenous grafts (AVG) are artificially created connections between the arteries and veins bypassing the capillary bed using a device (graft or synthetic tube) that is implanted under the skin at the site of the planned dialysis access. The implanted graft is used as the site for needle placement and access during hemodialysis. Unlike AVF, AVG do not need to mature; therefore, the delay between placement and first use is usually significantly shorter—often around 2–3 weeks. The procedure for graft placement is performed primarily by vascular surgeons, frequently as an outpatient procedure. The most common type of graft used is a polytetrafluoroethylene (PTFE) graft. AVG are primarily placed in patients who are unable to undergo AVF formation due to anatomical issues, peripheral vascular disease, or other medical comorbidities. Arteriovenous grafts have higher risk of infection than AVF due to the synthetic material used in the graft.

AVG Type and Location

- Forearm: radial artery-basilic vein graft.
- Forearm: brachial artery-basilic vein graft.
- Upper arm: brachial artery-axillary vein graft.
- Thigh: femoral artery-femoral vein graft.

AVF Versus AVG

There are several key differences between AVF and AVG that need to be considered when selecting the ideal permanent dialysis access type for a particular patient

- AVF are made entirely of native materials and require high-quality vessels in close proximity to each other that can be anastomosed.
- AVF may be less effective than AVG in patients with peripheral vascular disease or veins with large collateral networks reducing direct flow.
- AVF have significantly longer maturation time (6–8 weeks up to multiple months or a year) compared to AVG (2–3 weeks).
- AVG have increased risk of thrombosis and infection relative to AVF.
- Current NKF KDOQI clinical practice guidelines have established a recommended sequence of dialysis access types and anatomic locations and have suggested that forearm and upper arm AVF are preferred in ascending anatomical position from wrist to elbow, followed by synthetic grafts (AVG) placed in the forearm or upper arm.

Outcomes and Complications with AVF and AVG [1, 6]

Dialysis access dysfunction can be characterized by the type of failure and complications occurring. Clinical examination of AVG includes visual inspection of the area for bleeding, bruising, extremity swelling, or signs of infection including fever, local erythema, swelling, drainage, or tenderness. The dialysis access site should be palpated for thrills and pulsations as well as overall dialysis access characterization of diameter and compressibility. Thrills are common in mature well-functioning AVG over the arterial anastomosis, while pulsatility is usually an indicator of occlusion; changes in thrill or pulsatility may also indicate dialysis access dysfunction.

An understanding of the causes of different types of failure helps identify the type of intervention required in order to maintain effective dialysis access. A summary of the types of dialysis access failure and their common causes is listed in Table 15.2. Dialysis access failure may result from one or more of these causes and in some cases has a multifactorial etiology.

Common complications of AVF and AVG dialysis accesses include:

- Infection.
- Thrombosis.
- Stenosis (possible arterial, graft, venous, or central locations).
- Pseudoaneurysm (AVG) or aneurysm (AVF).

Table 15.2 Dialysis access failure type, definition, and cause, based on the SIR dysfunctional access guidelines [1]

Failure	Definition	Causes of failure
Anatomic	Failure due to anatomic structure variability around the dialysis access site, in particular arterial and venous abnormalities	1. Venous or intragraft stenosis within synthetic grafts 2. Venous drainage system or anastomotic site stenosis of native fistula access 3. Central venous stenosis 4. Intragraft stenosis or stenosis of the matured hypertrophied venous segment of the AVF 5. Excess collateral venous drainage preventing AVF maturation 6. Arterial stenosis proximal to dialysis access 7. Compression from extrinsic sources causing dialysis dysfunction
Physiologic	Failure (due to thrombosis) resulting from processes which are biological, chemical, or mechanical in nature and have no discernible anatomical cause	1. Hypercoagulable state leading to stenosis and dialysis access occlusion 2. Low cardiac output states reducing rate of flow through dialysis access

- Non-maturation (AVF).
- Ischemia.

  Non-maturation has been reported to occur in 25–30% of all AVF created [7].

Fistulograms and Assessment of Access Function

Dialysis accesses should be assessed regularly by clinicians for indicators of dysfunction. Any changes to clinical exam findings, hemodynamic variables, or increased suspicion of dialysis access dysfunction between visits should be followed up with further investigation including fistulograms or duplex ultrasonography of dialysis access [1]:

- Fistulogram: (diagnostic angiogram/venogram) involves the use of fluoroscopic tools for visualization of the dialysis access from proximal arterial component through anastomosis or prosthetic graft and into venous collecting systems.

  Depending on the type of dysfunction, further proximal arterial system or central venous imaging may be required (Fig. 15.1).
- Duplex ultrasonography: the use of color Doppler ultrasound to image the flow within a dialysis access and characterize the patency as well as any changes observed on a clinical exam.

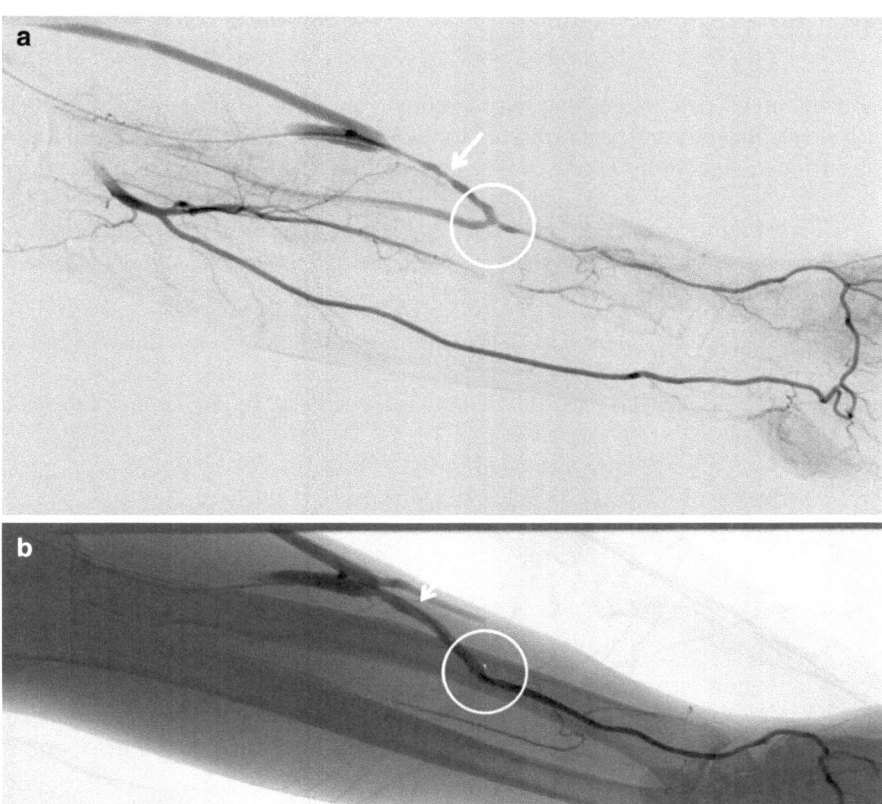

Fig. 15.1 (**a**) Fistulogram of radiocephalic fistula (circle) with functionally significant stenosis (solid arrow). (**b**) Fistulogram of radiocephalic fistula with satisfactory angiographic result following balloon angioplasty of functionally significant stenosis

Preoperative Evaluation

Given the superior outcomes of AVF vs. AVG, it is becoming common practice to evaluate the venous and arterial networks pre-AVF/AVG placement via color Doppler ultrasound [8].

Although angiography traditionally has been considered the gold standard for evaluation of vascular networks, ultrasonography is increasingly being recognized for its utility in providing superior information on morphology of the vasculature [8]. Further, it is a noninvasive method without need for contrast in individuals with pre-existing declining renal function and risk of nephrotoxicity [8].

Dialysis Access Patency

Interventional radiologists play an important role in the management of dialysis access dysfunction and patency issues using percutaneous procedures. An outline of the different definitions used to define patency based on interventions required and complications resulting based on the SIR guidelines [1] is presented in Table 15.3.

Understanding patency definitions for dialysis accesses is important for the assessment of long-term effectiveness of dialysis access and the benefits of intervention.

Indications for interventions include [1]

1. Dialysis access stenosis of >50% luminal diameter with clinical signs of dysfunction.
2. Central vein stenosis of >50% luminal diameter and graft hemodynamically compromised.
3. Non-maturing AVF after extended period of time.
4. Thrombosis of dialysis access leading to access dysfunction.

Factors Affecting Dialysis Access Patency

Considering the superior clinical outcomes associated with hemodialysis AVF formation prior to RRT, it is important to consider factors which may impact patency of a dialysis access site, so that clinicians can prophylactically choose the appropriate mode of access [9].

Patient factors impacting on the patency of a dialysis access site include a variety of comorbid conditions affecting the vascular system such as

- Increasing age and decreasing elasticity of the blood vessels.
- Risk factors causing endothelial dysfunction such as smoking, lipid dysregulation, and sub-optimal diet.

Table 15.3 Definitions of patency based on the SIR dysfunctional access management guidelines [1]

Patency type	Definition
Primary	The period during which the dialysis access remains patent without intervention prior to thrombosis or stenosis event occurring and re-intervention is required. Re-intervention of any region within the access circuit ends the primary patency period
Assisted primary	The period during which dialysis access remains patent and patency is maintained through interventions until the dialysis access becomes thrombosed and thrombolysis or thrombectomy is required
Secondary	The period from dialysis access creation until surgical declotting, revision of access, or abandonment of access
Cumulative	The total period during which the access remains patent, including all primary interventions, thrombectomy, and thrombolysis procedures

- Systemic medical conditions such as diabetes mellitus and peripheral vascular disease.
- Anatomically small-caliber vessels with no identifiable cause [9].

Interventions

Percutaneous Transluminal Angioplasty

Percutaneous transluminal angioplasty (PTA) is indicated as first-line treatment for dialysis access and central venous stenosis [1, 10]. PTA may be used in non-maturing fistulas on the anastomosis site in order to increase inflow to the maturing arteriovenous connection. PTA involves puncturing the dialysis access site and deploying a 6–8 mm balloon in order to dilate the lumen and remove the stenosis. The balloon is inflated and remains in place for 30 s and then is deflated. The dialysis access and surrounding vessels are imaged under fluoroscopy to evaluate the stenosis and determine whether additional intervention is needed.

Contraindications include

- Absolute contraindications—access site infection.
- Relative contraindications—contrast allergy, severe metabolic dysfunction requiring immediate dialysis.

PTA can also be used after thrombectomy or thrombolysis to treat underlying stenosis in patients with thrombosed dialysis access. Studies have suggested that treatment of significant stenosis will reduce rates of dialysis access thrombosis and improve patency rates (Table 15.4) [11–25].

Table 15.4 Success and patency rates reported in the literature for AVF and AVG following PTA [11–24]

	Access type	Reported rates (%)
Clinical success	AVF	86–100
Clinical success	AVG	85–100
6-month primary patency	AVF	25–95
6-month primary patency	AVG	31–61
12-month primary patency	AVF	34–62
12-month primary patency	AVG	20–41
12-month secondary patency	AVF	67–86

Endoluminal Stent Placement

Endoluminal stent placement is indicated as first-line treatment for pseudoaneu-rysms, venous rupture resulting from PTA, and surgically inaccessible veins with stenosis (Table 15.5) [1, 6, 10, 26–31]. Stents may be deployed after PTA for [1]:

- Peripheral stenosis with failed balloon angioplasty, difficult surgical access, or contraindication to surgery.
- Central venous stenosis with failed balloon angioplasty or recurred within 3 months of successful PTA.
- Post-PTA outflow vein rupture.
- Note: stents should not be deployed at the access sites.

The procedure for endoluminal stent placement involves obtaining endovascular access, characterizing the dialysis access vasculature under fluoroscopy, and deploy-ing a stent after balloon inflation at the site of stenosis. Common stents used include bare metal stents (BMS), polytetrafluoroethylene (PTFE) grafts, and heparin-coated stents.

Contraindications include

- Absolute contraindications—access site infection.
- Relative contraindications—contrast allergy, severe metabolic dysfunction requiring immediate dialysis.

Table 15.5 Success and patency rates reported in the literature for AVF and AVG following stent placement [6, 26–31]

	Access type	Reported rates (%)
Clinical success	AVF	92–100
Clinical success	AVG	88–100
6-month primary patency	AVF	39–94
6-month primary patency	AVG	11–87
12-month primary patency	AVF	31–94
12-month primary patency	AVG	19–61
12-month secondary patency	AVF	82–94
12-month secondary patency	AVG	48–100

Chemical (Pharmacologic) Thrombolysis and Mechanical Thrombectomy

Thrombosis with or without associated vessel stenosis is a common cause of dialysis access dysfunction in both AVF and AVG accesses [25, 32, 33]. Management of thrombosed dialysis accesses may include pharmacologic thrombolysis, where urokinase, reteplase (r-PA recombinant plasminogen activator), or alteplase (rt-PA recombinant tissue plasminogen activator) is injected locally in the thrombosed dialysis access or mechanical thrombectomy whereby mechanical devices are used endovascularly. Primary patency rates tend to be higher following surgical procedures, and vessel re-occlusion due to thrombosis is seen less frequently [34] (Figs. 15.2 and 15.3).

Contraindications for pharmacologic thrombolysis include:

- Recent surgery.
- Gastrointestinal hemorrhage or increased risk of bleeding.
- Patients with hemoptysis.
- Patients with intracranial tumors.

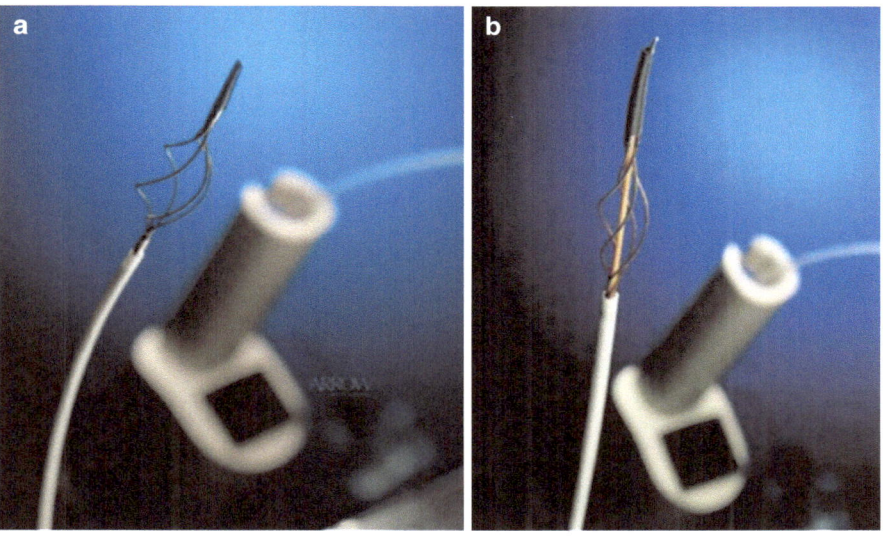

Fig. 15.2 (**a**) 5 French Arrow-Trerotola™ percutaneous thrombolytic device (PTD). (**b**) 7 French over-the-wire Arrow-Trerotola™ PTD for thrombectomy. (Reprinted with permission of Teleflex Inc.)

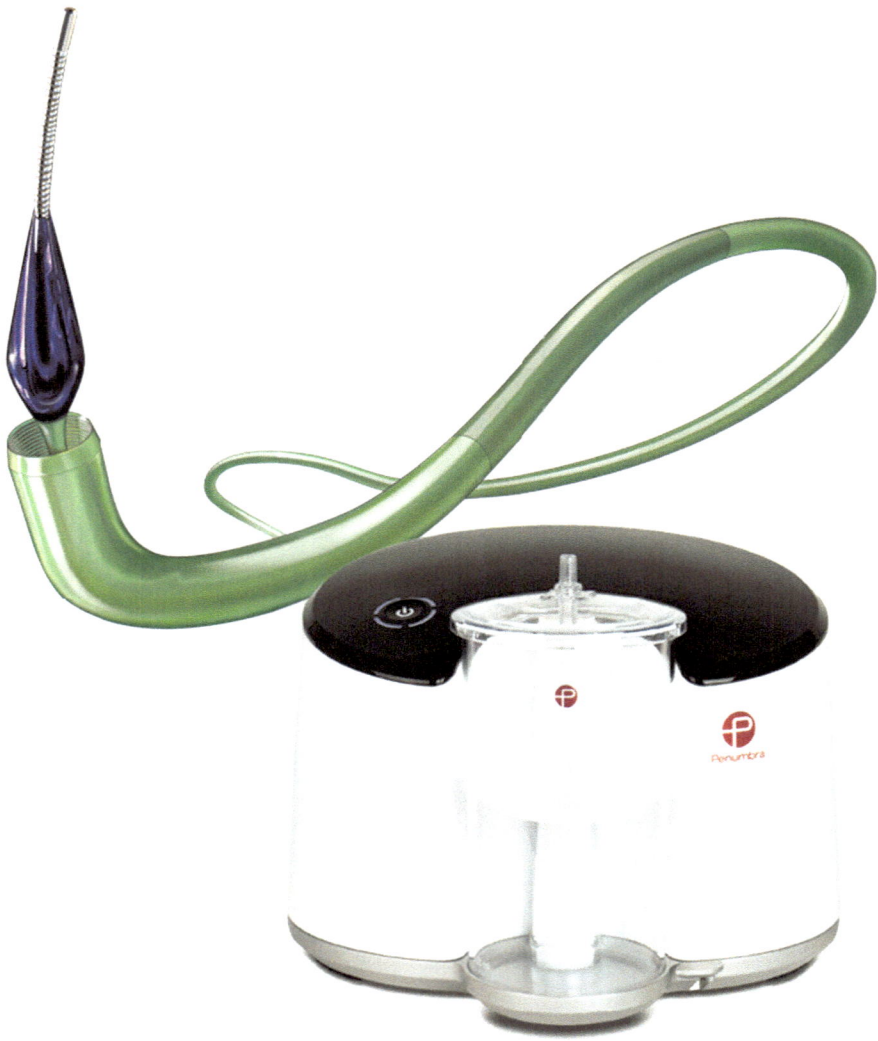

Fig. 15.3 Indigo CAT D™ percutaneous thrombolytic device (PTD). (Reprinted with permission of Penumbra Inc.)

In addition, some centers utilize a combined pharmacomechanical thrombectomy approach, whereby devices that can macerate clots are used in addition to local urokinase or tPA injection. Patency rates following thrombolysis and thrombectomy reported in the literature are outlined in Table 15.6 [35–44].

	Access type	Reported rates (%)
Table 15.6 Success and patency rates reported in the literature for AVF and AVG following thrombolysis and thrombectomy [35–44]		
Clinical success	AVF	55–100
Clinical success	AVG	53–100
6-month primary patency	AVF	20–80
6-month primary patency	AVG	28–72
12-month primary patency	AVF	19–58
12-month primary patency	AVG	17–58
12-month secondary patency	AVF	74–92
12-month secondary patency	AVG	35–96

Collateral Vessel Embolization

One of the causes of non-maturing arteriovenous fistulas is an extensive collateral venous collection and drainage system, which reduces the pressure load on the anastomotic vein reducing the rate of fistula maturation. Interventions for non-maturing arteriovenous fistulas include PTA of the anastomosis to increase venous inflow and collateral vessel embolization to increase venous pressure. Collateral vessels may be managed through surgical ligation or endovascular embolization [7].

The procedure for collateral vessel embolization involves a clinical assessment of the dialysis access area and characterization of the target vein as well as collateral vasculature, after which a catheter is threaded through the dialysis access and placed in the collateral veins, where embolization material (usually coils) is deployed until vessels are occluded [7].

Summary

Currently, arteriovenous fistulas are indicated as first-line treatment for permanent dialysis access creation due to reduced rates of complications; however, AVG are indicated in patients with shorter life expectancy requiring immediate dialysis or currently undergoing dialysis through a central catheter.

Interventional radiologists play an important role in the objective assessment of dialysis access function through the use of fistulograms and in the maintenance of functional dialysis accesses through percutaneous interventional procedures.

The evolution of dialysis access interventional procedures has extended the life span of permanent dialysis accesses and improved outcomes for patients undergoing hemodialysis, reducing the need for creation of alternative dialysis access sites.

Current procedures including PTA, stent placement, and pharmacologic or mechanical thrombolysis help maintain dialysis access patency. Percutaneous and endovascular interventions are first-line treatment for maintenance of access patency due to low morbidity and comparable outcomes to surgical revision and intervention.

Acknowledgment We would like to thank Dr. Lazar Milovanovic for his contributions to this chapter (information given on first page of chapter).

References

1. Aruny JE, Lewis CA, Cardella JF, et al. Quality improvement guidelines for percutaneous management of the thrombosed or dysfunctional dialysis access. J Vasc Interv Radiol. 2003;14:S247–53.
2. Brescia MJ, Cimino JE, Appel K, Hurwich BJ. Chronic hemodialysis using venipuncture and a surgically created arteriovenous fistula. N Engl J Med. 1966;275(20):1089–92.
3. Wasse H. Place of percutaneous fistula devices in contemporary management of vascular access. Clin J Am Soc Nephrol. 2019;14(6):938–40.
4. Robbin ML, Chamberlain NE, Lockhart ME, Gallichio MH, Young CJ, Deierhoi MH, Allon M. Hemodialysis arteriovenous fistula maturity: US evaluation. Radiology. 2002;225(1):59–64.
5. Vascular Access 2006 Work Group. Clinical practice guidelines for vascular access. Am J Kidney Dis. 2006;48(Suppl 1):S176–247.
6. Haskal ZJ, Trerotola S, Dolmatch B, et al. Stent graft versus balloon angioplasty for failing dialysis-access grafts. N Engl J Med. 2010;362:494–503.
7. Zangan SM, Falk A. Optimizing arteriovenous fistula maturation. Semin Interv Radiol. 2009;26(2):144–50.
8. Wiese P, Nonnast-Daniel B. Colour Doppler ultrasound in dialysis access. Nephrol Dial Transplant. 2004;19(8):1956–63.
9. Smith GE, Gohil R, Chetter IC. Factors affecting the patency of arteriovenous fistulas for dialysis access. J Vasc Surg. 2012;55(3):849–55.
10. Bittl JA. Catheter interventions for hemodialysis fistulas and grafts. J Am Coll Cardiol Interv. 2010;3(1):1–11.
11. Aftab SA, Tay KH, Irani FG, Gong Lo RH, Gogna A, Haaland B, Tan BS. Randomized clinical trial of cutting balloon angioplasty versus high-pressure balloon angioplasty in hemodialysis arteriovenous fistula stenoses resistant to conventional balloon angioplasty. J Vasc Interv Radiol. 2014;25(2):190–8.
12. Clark TW, Cohen RA, Kwak A, Markmann JF, Stavropoulos SW, Patel AA, Trerotola SO. Salvage of nonmaturing native fistulas by using angioplasty. Radiology. 2007;242(1):286–92.
13. Katsanos K, Karnabatidis D, Kitrou P, Spiliopoulos S, Christeas N, Siablis D. Paclitaxel-coated balloon angioplasty vs. plain balloon dilation for the treatment of failing dialysis access: 6-month interim results from a prospective randomized controlled trial. J Endovasc Ther. 2012;19(2):263–72.
14. Kim WS, Pyun WB, Kang BC. The primary patency of percutaneous transluminal angioplasty in hemodialysis patients with vascular access failure. Korean Circ J. 2011;41(9):512–7.
15. Maeda K, Furukawa A, Yamasaki M, Murata K. Percutaneous transluminal angioplasty for Brescia-Cimino hemodialysis fistula dysfunction: technical success rate, patency rate and factors that influence the results. Eur J Radiol. 2005;54(3):426–30.
16. Manninen HI, Kaukanen E, Mäkinen K, Karhapää P. Endovascular salvage of nonmaturing autogenous hemodialysis fistulas: comparison with endovascular therapy of failing mature fistulas. J Vasc Interv Radiol. 2008;19(6):870–6.

17. Rajan DK, Bunston S, Misra S, Pinto R, Lok CE. Dysfunctional autogenous hemodialysis fistulas: outcomes after angioplasty—are there clinical predictors of patency? Radiology. 2004;232(2):508–15.
18. Veroux P, Giaquinta A, Tallarita T, Sinagra N, Virgilio C, Zerbo D, Veroux M. Primary balloon angioplasty of small (≤2 mm) cephalic veins improves primary patency of arteriovenous fistulae and decreases reintervention rates. J Vasc Surg. 2013;57(1):131–6.
19. Beathard GA. Percutaneous transvenous angioplasty in the treatment of vascular access stenosis. Kidney Int. 1992;42(6):1390–7.
20. Kanterman RY, Vesely TM, Pilgram TK, Guy BW, Windus DW, Picus D. Dialysis access grafts: anatomic location of venous stenosis and results of angioplasty. Radiology. 1995;195(1):135.
21. Lai CC, Chung HM, Tsai HL, Mar GY, Tseng CJ, Liu CP. Intragraft pressures predict outcomes in hemodialysis patients with graft outflow lesions undergoing percutaneous transluminal angioplasty. Catheter Cardiovasc Interv. 2010;76(2):206–11.
22. Mori Y, Horikawa K, Sato K, Mimuro N, Toriyama T, Kawahara H. Stenotic lesions in vascular access: treatment with transluminal angioplasty using high-pressure balloons. Intern Med (Tokyo, Japan). 1994;33(5):284–7.
23. Safa AA, Valji K, Roberts AC, Ziegler TW, Hye RJ, Oglevie SB. Detection and treatment of dysfunctional hemodialysis access grafts: effect of a surveillance program on graft patency and the incidence of thrombosis. Radiology. 1996;199(3):653–7.
24. Vesely TM, Siegel JB. Use of the peripheral cutting balloon to treat hemodialysis-related stenoses. J Vasc Interv Radiol. 2005;16(12):1593–603.
25. Van Ha T. Percutaneous management of thrombosed dialysis access grafts. Semin Interv Radiol. 2004;21(2):77–81.
26. Vesely TM, Amin MZ, Pilgram T. Use of stents and stent grafts to salvage angioplasty failures in patients with hemodialysis grafts. Semin Dial. 2008;21(1):100–4.
27. Chan MR, Bedi S, Sanchez RJ, et al. Stent placement versus angioplasty improves patency of arteriovenous grafts and blood flow of arteriovenous fistula. Clin J Am Soc Nephrol. 2008;3(3):699–705.
28. Kolakowski S Jr, Dougherty MJ, Calligaro KD. Salvaging prosthetic dialysis fistulas with stents: forearm versus upper arm grafts. J Vasc Surg. 2003;38(4):719–23.
29. Dolmatch BL, Duch JM, Winder R, et al. Salvage of angioplasty failures and complications in hemodialysis arteriovenous access using the FLUENCY plus stent graft: technical and 180-day patency results. J Vasc Interv Radiol. 2012;23(4):478–87.
30. Jones RG, Willis AP, Jones C, McCafferty IJ, Riley PL. Long-term results of stent-graft placement to treat central venous stenosis and occlusion in hemodialysis patients with arteriovenous fistulas. J Vasc Interv Radiol. 2011;22(9):1240–5.
31. Kim YC, Won JY, Choi SY, et al. Percutaneous treatment of central venous stenosis in hemodialysis patients: long-term outcomes. Cardiovasc Intervent Radiol. 2009;32(2):271–8.
32. Bush RL, Lin PH, Lumsden AB. Management of thrombosed dialysis access: thrombectomy versus thrombolysis. Semin Vasc Surg. 2004;17(1):32–9.
33. Mendez-Castillo A, Hassain S, Castaneda F. Pharmacomechanical thrombolysis of dialysis access grafts using the MTI Castaneda over-the-wire brush catheter and reteplase. Semin Interv Radiol. 2004;21(2):129–34.
34. Green LD, Lee DS, Kucey DS. A metaanalysis comparing surgical thrombectomy, mechanical thrombectomy, and pharmacomechanical thrombolysis for thrombosed dialysis grafts. J Vasc Surg. 2002;36(5):939–45.
35. Jain G, Maya ID, Allon M. Outcomes of percutaneous mechanical thrombectomy of arteriovenous fistulas in hemodialysis patients. Semin Dial. 2008;21(6):581–3.
36. Littler P, Cullen N, Gould D, Bakran A, Powell S. AngioJet thrombectomy for occluded dialysis fistula: outcome data. Cardiovasc Intervent Radiol. 2009;32(2):265–70.
37. Kakkos SK, Haddad GK, Haddad J, Scully MM. Percutaneous rheolytic thrombectomy for thrombosed autogenous fistula and prosthetic arteriovenous grafts: outcome after aggressive surveillance and endovascular management. J Endovasc Ther. 2008;15(1):91–102.

38. Bakken AM, Galaria II, Agerstrand C, et al. Percutaneous therapy to maintain dialysis access successfully prolongs functional duration after primary failure. Ann Vasc Surg. 2007;21(4):474–80.
39. Rabin I, Shani M, Peer A, et al. Effect of timing of thrombectomy on survival of thrombosed arteriovenous hemodialysis grafts. Vasc Endovascular Surg. 2013;47(5):342–5.
40. Uflacker R, Rajagopalan PR, Selby JB, Hannegan C. Thrombosed dialysis access grafts: randomized comparison of the Amplatz thrombectomy device and surgical thromboembolectomy. Eur Radiol. 2004;14(11):2009–14.
41. Sofocleous CT, Hinrichs CR, Weiss SH, et al. Alteplase for hemodialysis access graft thrombolysis. J Vasc Interv Radiol. 2002;13(8):775–84.
42. Barth KH, Gosnell MR, Palestrant AM, et al. Hydrodynamic thrombectomy system versus pulse-spray thrombolysis for thrombosed hemodialysis grafts: a multicenter prospective randomized comparison. Radiology. 2000;217(3):678–84.
43. Smits HF, Smits JH, Wust AF, Buskens E, Blankenstijn PJ. Percutaneous thrombolysis of thrombosed haemodialysis access grafts: comparison of three mechanical devices. Nephrol Dial Transplant. 2002;17(3):467–73.
44. Vogel PM, Bansal V, Marshall MW. Thrombosed hemodialysis grafts: lyse and wait with tissue plasminogen activator or urokinase compared to mechanical thrombolysis with the Arrow-Trerotola percutaneous thrombolytic device. J Vasc Interv Radiol. 2001;12(10):1157–65.

Chapter 16
Interventional Radiology in Women's Health

Anne-Sophie Fortier and Lazar Milovanovic

Uterine Leiomyoma (Fibroid) Embolization (UFE)

The primary method of management of uterine leiomyoma was hysterectomy or myomectomy or medical measures prior to the development of uterine fibroid embolization (UFE) as an interventional procedure. UFE was first performed by Jean Jacques Merland and colleagues in 1989 with subsequent publication of results in 1995 [1]. UFE initially intended as a treatment for pelvic hemorrhage and has been used for symptomatic leiomyomas since 1995 [2].

Definitions

- Leiomyoma: benign tumor of smooth muscle containing fibrous connective tissue also referred to as a "fibroid" or a "myoma."
- Embolization: the obstruction or occlusion of a vessel through the infusion of an embolic agent resulting in reduced blood flow distal to the embolized area.
- Submucosal leiomyoma: located beneath the mucosal lining and may protrude or be adjacent to uterine cavity.
- Subserosal leiomyoma: located under the uterine serosa—does not protrude into uterine cavity but may alter shape of outer surface of uterus.
- Pedunculated leiomyoma: having a stalk by which the leiomyoma is attached to the uterus.

A.-S. Fortier (✉) · L. Milovanovic
Michael G. DeGroote School of Medicine,
McMaster University, Hamilton, ON, Canada
e-mail: annesophie.fortier@medportal.ca; lazar.milovanovic@medportal.ca

© The Author(s), under exclusive license to Springer Nature
Switzerland AG 2022
S. Athreya, M. Albahhar (eds.), *Demystifying Interventional Radiology*,
https://doi.org/10.1007/978-3-031-12023-7_16

Epidemiology

Uterine leiomyomas are the most common benign tumor of the female genitourinary tract [3]. Studies report that 25% of women of reproductive age are affected by uterine leiomyomas with Afro-Caribbean populations experiencing higher prevalence and disease burden [3]. Reported prevalence of uterine leiomyomas is greater than 80% in African-American women and 70% in white women by the age of 50 [4]. Proportion of leiomyomas that are symptomatic ranges from 20 to 50% [3], and common presenting symptoms include pelvic and back pain, urinary or bowel obstruction, dyspareunia, infertility, and miscarriage [2, 5, 6].

Indications/Contraindications

UFE is an elective procedure performed on premenopausal women with confirmed uterine leiomyoma who have undergone tests to rule out other pathologies such as endometrial carcinoma [1]. The primary aim for intervention in patients with uterine leiomyoma is quality of life improvement and symptom relief [5]. For these reasons, asymptomatic fibroids are not an indication to undergo UFE [4]. Pedunculated subserosal fibroids are a relative contraindication for UFE and are primarily managed through hysterectomy or myomectomy due to the high risk of complications [5].

UFE is not usually performed in postmenopausal women since uterine fibroids generally decrease in size or regress without intervention after menopause. This is attributed to the hormone dependence of these fibroids [7].

Patients who are considering future pregnancy should be counseled appropriately as there is insufficient current data for prospective studies evaluating conception in women post-UFE [5]. While noting that successful pregnancies have occurred following UFE, myomectomy is currently the standard of care over UFE for patients with plans to conceive in the future [2, 8].

Absolute contraindications for UFE are viable pregnancy, active infection, and suspected malignancy in the uterus, cervix, or the ovaries and fallopian tubes [8].

Pre-Procedure Patient Work-Up

The pre-procedure patient work-up includes the use of laboratory tests and diagnostic imaging to assess patients for pre-existing conditions and fully characterize the uterine fibroid prior to intervention (Fig. 16.1).

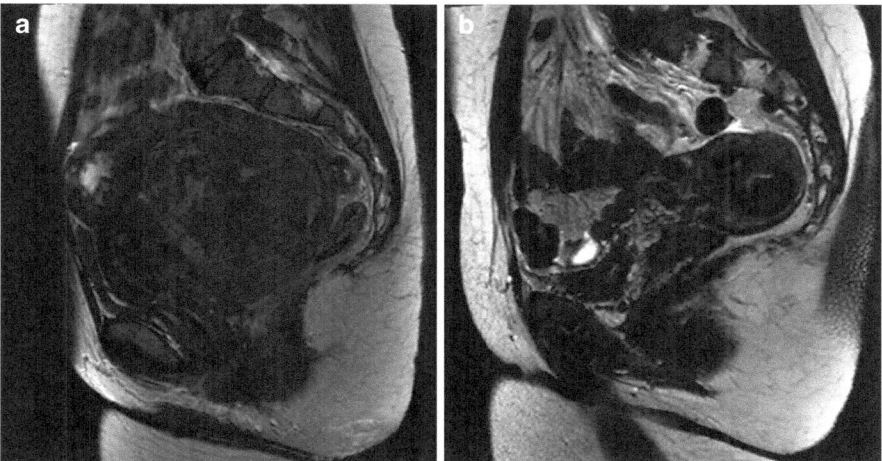

Fig. 16.1 (**a**) Large myometrial fibroid before uterine artery embolization. (**b**) 9-month post-uterine artery embolization showing significant decrease in fibroid size and complete avascular necrosis

Laboratory Tests

- Complete blood count (CBC): allows interventional radiologist to screen patient for anemia and thrombocytopenia.
- Coagulation studies: coagulation studies are indicated in patients with history of liver disease or anticoagulant therapy or high index of suspicion but are not required for all patients undergoing UFE.
- Thyroid-stimulating hormone (TSH): allows interventional radiologist to rule out hypothyroidism as a cause of excessive vaginal bleeding [2].

Diagnostic Imaging

In general, the goal of diagnostic imaging in the pre-procedure setting is to confirm the diagnosis of fibroids and then assess characteristics of these fibroids including the size, location, and number of fibroids. Imaging is also used to assess the patient's pelvic vasculature including the specific blood fibroid blood supply and to detect any other pathologies that may be present and need to be ruled out, such as endometrial mass and adenomyosis. The main diagnostic imaging modalities used in the pre-procedure settings are pelvic ultrasound (USS) and contrast-enhanced magnetic resonance (MR) imaging.

Ultrasound

USS is the gold standard for pre-procedure diagnostic imaging assessment of fibroids [9]. In addition to being minimally invasive, it is also a readily available and inexpensive option. However, it is operator-dependent and provides inferior anatomical characterization relative to MRI. It is not effective for detection of adenomyosis or assessment of pelvic and fibroid vascularity.

Performing USS with a transvaginal approach is most useful; however, an abdominal USS may be required for visualization of an enlarged uterus. Other types of USS are saline-infusion sonohysterography, three-dimensional USS, and color Doppler USS [9].

Contrast-Enhanced MRI

Contrast-enhanced MRI offers more accurate and precise determination of fibroid location and characteristics compared to USS. It is an effective diagnostic imaging modality for detecting adenomyosis and characterizing pelvic anatomy. Gadolinium contrast is used to enhance vasculature. MRI can be used to determine tissue perfusion and assess fibroid infarction pre- and post-embolization. However, MRI is expensive and is not as widely available as USS. Contraindications to MRI include morbid obesity, claustrophobia, presence of defibrillators, and gadolinium contrast allergy [2].

Magnetic resonance angiography (MRA) is used for treatment planning in patients to assess the anatomical vasculature and determine interventional approach. Patients identified to have ovarian artery supply to their uterine fibroid(s) on MRA have a higher risk of treatment failure [10]. Assessment of blood supply can be an important predictor of treatment success: fibroids with high signal in T1-weighted images have been shown to have worse prognosis after UFE, while high signal in T2-weighted images prior to treatment has been shown to improve prognosis after UFE [11].

Pre-Treatment Patient Information

Prior to the procedure, it is a standard practice to bring the patient in for an initial clinical consult to go over the procedure, expectations, complications, and alternatives. The initial clinical consult serves as a forum to outline periprocedural medication and pain relief as well as symptoms of post-embolization syndrome. Finally, it provides the interventional radiologist an opportunity to go over the follow-up procedure with the patient and ensure that a plan has been made for the post-procedure clinical management and future follow-up.

Procedure Overview

Vascular Access

The patient is prepared and draped in a sterile fashion and placed under conscious sedation for the procedure [12]. Catheterization is usually initiated unilaterally or bilaterally through the common femoral arteries under fluoroscopic guidance [5]. Bilateral femoral arterial access is only utilized in some centers and may require two operators. It has been suggested that the bilateral femoral artery approach reduces patient radiation dose [13].

Angiography

Flush aortography is usually not required but can be helpful in patients with abnormal arterial anatomy and in patients undergoing repeat UAE, to identify any collateral blood vessels supplying the fibroid (Fig. 16.2) [5].

The angiographic steps for embolization are as follows:

1. After obtaining femoral artery access, a catheter is negotiated into the contralateral iliac artery.
2. Using oblique and road map views on the contralateral side, the internal iliac artery is selected.
3. The anterior division of the internal iliac artery is located using an ipsilateral oblique view.
4. A microcatheter is threaded through into the uterine artery. The use of a microcatheter is important for the prevention of arteriospasm and to enable effective free flow-directed embolization.

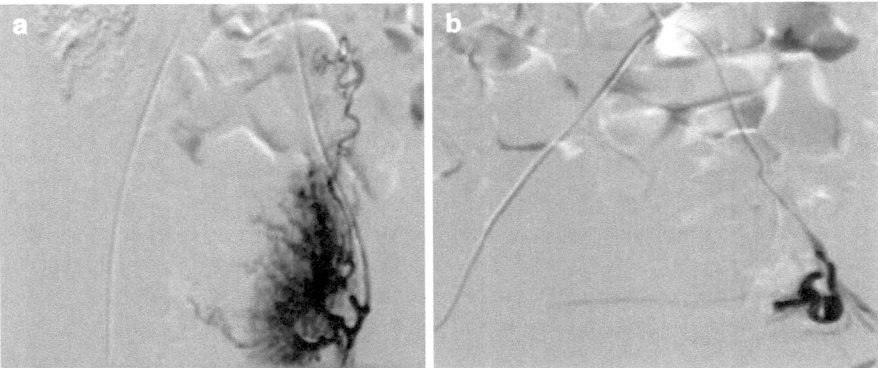

Fig. 16.2 (**a**) Left uterine artery angiogram pre-embolization for fibroid. (**b**) Left uterine artery angiogram post-embolization for fibroid

5. Once adequately positioned, the catheter is used to deploy an embolizing agent such as polyvinyl alcohol (PVA), Gelfoam, or calibrated trisacryl gelatin microspheres (CTGM) [12].
6. Using one of the angiographic end points (see next section), the uterine artery is embolized (Fig. 16.2b).
7. In order to produce adequate fibroid infarction, the uterine arteries need to be embolized bilaterally; therefore, the entire embolization process is then completed on the ipsilateral uterine artery

Angiographic Appearance

The uterine arteries are usually hypertrophied, tortuous, and laterally displaced. The angiographic end point refers to the angiographic sign used to determine when to cease embolization. There are multiple proposed end points that are currently used, and the exact end point remains controversial [5]. The common end points used by interventional radiologists today are:

1. Complete stasis of blood flow in the isolated artery over 5 or 10 cardiac beats.
2. Complete stasis of blood flow in the isolated artery with reflux back along angiographic catheter.
3. A "pruned tree" appearance (abrupt cut-off of multiple arterioles) while forward flow in the main uterine artery is maintained.

Immediate Complications

Immediate complications of UFE include thromboembolic events, infection, vascular access injuries, non-target embolization, and periprocedural pain and can be related to contrast agent use as well as the vascular access procedure [8, 12, 14, 15]. A common complication of UFE within the first 48 h after procedure is post-embolization syndrome, which is comprised of pelvic pain, nausea, vomiting, fever, general malaise, and transient leukocytosis; it can occur in up to 34% of patients [11, 15, 16]. Thromboembolic complications can include uterine ischemia, uterine necrosis, deep vein thrombosis, pulmonary embolus, and death [14, 15].

While the goal of UFE is to cause fibroid ischemia and necrosis, ischemia and necrosis may also occur acutely to the uterus and will often be associated with worsening pain; acute clinical and MRI follow-up is recommended in these patients [14]. Uterine necrosis is a rare, acute, major complication treated by urgent hysterectomy to prevent sepsis and death in patients [14].

Infectious complications can include endometritis and sepsis and may require intravenous antibiotics or surgery; differentiation from fever and leukocytosis during post-embolization syndrome is difficult; therefore, a high index of suspicion is required [14]. Death associated with UFE has been reported in the literature, with causes including pulmonary embolus, uterine necrosis, and sepsis with multiorgan failure [14]. Non-target embolization may result in soft tissue necrosis [14].

Delayed Complications

Delayed complications for UFE include transient or permanent amenorrhea and subsequent infertility, chronic vaginal discharge, transcervical fibroid expulsion, and premature menopause [2, 8, 12]. In some cases, delayed infection of necrotic dominant fibroids can occur in the weeks or months following UFE; these infections can result in sepsis and may require myomectomy or hysterectomy [14]. Several studies have assessed pregnancy outcomes after UAE with or without comparison to alternative treatments and have found increased risk of spontaneous abortion, malpresentation, and delivery via caesarean section after UFE [8]. Other complications include sciatic nerve injury leading to buttock claudication [2].

Outcomes

The success of uterine fibroid embolization is determined by assessing the change in volume of the fibroid as well as the uterus on MRI along with symptomatic improvement on patient history [8]. Post-procedure MRI is recommended at 3-month intervals for evaluation of fibroid volume and tissue characteristics on weighted imaging, with initial fibroid infarction occurring as early as 24 h after UFE [12, 17]. On T1-weighted MRIs, the degeneration and devascularization of fibroids can be observed as increased signal density, while the same results on T2-weighted MRIs will be visualized as decreased signals [2]. Fibroid volume is expected to continue decreasing for over 1 year with increasing symptom improvement [2].

Compared to other uterine-sparing therapies, uterine fibroid embolization holds several advantages and disadvantages with regard to post-procedure outcomes. There is little difference in complication rates, symptom severity scores, and miscarriage rates following UFE when compared to surgical myomectomy [17]. There is sparse and conflicting data on pregnancy rates post-UFE; a 2021 systematic review found that patients have higher conception rates post-myomectomy, but further research is needed to explore this association [18]. UFE is linked to a shorter recovery time, but also has a higher rate of treatment failure than myomectomies [17]. The opposite scenario is encountered when considering MRI-guided high-intensity focused ultrasound (HIFU) for uterine fibroids. While associated with increased severity of post-procedure pain and a slower recovery time compared to MRI-guided HIFU, UFE tends to provide better symptomatic relief and has lower rates of treatment failure [17].

Treatment Failure

Treatment failure presents in patients as regrowth of fibroids and residual viable fibroid on imaging indicating incomplete fibroid infarction. Failure is defined as reintervention through subsequent hysterectomy, definitive myomectomy, or repeat embolization; it can also present as failure of symptom improvement at long-term patient follow-up [14]. There are multiple possible causes of treatment failure in UFE including incomplete embolization of the uterine artery, arterial spasm, recanalization of the embolized arteries, extensive non-uterine artery collateral supply, and effects from gonadotropin agonists [14]. The location of fibroids within the uterus also influences the rate of treatment failure; cervical fibroids have poorer vascularity compared to other sites and reach complete infraction in only 20% of cases [17]. Additionally, the lower segment of the uterus and the front wall of the uterus are locations where UFE failure appears to occur more commonly. Contradictory evidence exists on differences in infarction rates between serosal and transmural fibroids [17]. The concept of location-dependent treatment success for uterine fibroid embolization is incompletely characterized and requires further investigation to elucidate.

Collateral arterial supply to a fibroid from a source other than the uterine arteries is an important cause of treatment failure in UFE. This source is usually the ovarian arteries as 4–8% of cases involve some level of collateral ovarian arterial supply to the fibroids [19]. Measures used to mitigate this risk include the use of magnetic resonance angiography (MRA) pre-UFE and non-contrast cone beam CT to characterize the fibroids' arterial flow post-UFE [17, 19, 20]. Further investigative and treatment decisions, including ovarian artery catheterization, can then be made based on the information provided by the imaging [20]. These modalities can help avoid incomplete fibroid infarction and reduce the rate of reintervention necessary following UFE.

As detailed above, reintervention rates following UFE are consistently higher than following myomectomy, but these rates vary by study. A 2012 randomized controlled trial demonstrated a 14% reintervention rate post-UFE compared to 2.7% post-myomectomy 2 years after the procedure [18]. Another 2018 longitudinal retrospective cohort study had a reintervention rate of 4% for myomectomy and 7% for UFE 1 year later. The 5-year rate increased to 19% and 24%, respectively [21]. These findings continue to hold true, as a 2021 systemic review found the reintervention rate post-UFE to be 4% higher than post-myomectomy in studies with 3 years of follow-up [22].

Postpartum Hemorrhage

Definition and Epidemiology

Postpartum hemorrhage (PPH) is the loss of more than 500 mL of blood following vaginal delivery or more than 1000 mL of blood following caesarean section. It can also be defined by a reduction of 10% or more in the patient's hematocrit and is considered an obstetric emergency [12]. Patients experiencing PPH will usually remain asymptomatic until they have lost more than 2000 mL of blood, at which point clinical signs of hypovolemia may be present [23]. PPH is classified by the temporal relationship of onset with delivery; primary PPH occurs within 24 h of delivery, while secondary PPH occurs between 6- and 12-week postpartum period [24, 25]. PPH occurs in 2–11% of deliveries [26] and is currently the main worldwide cause of pregnancy-related death [27]. Maternal death risk from PPH is estimated to be 1 per 1000 deliveries [28].

Etiology of PPH

The etiologies of PPH can be remembered by the 4 T mnemonic: tone (uterine atony, loss of uterine muscle tone resulting in decompression of vessels), trauma (lacerations, uterine rupture, hematoma), tissue (retained products of conception, invasive placenta), and thrombin (inherited coagulopathy). PPH may be categorized as a primary (occurring less than 24 h after delivery) or secondary (occurring more than 24 h after delivery) [29]. Causes of primary PPH include atony, lacerations, uterine rupture, and coagulopathies [30]. Causes of secondary PPH include subinvolution of placental site and subsequent atony, retained products of conception, infection, and inherited coagulation defects [30].

Preliminary Management

The therapeutic target for patients experiencing PPH is to terminate the bleeding early enough to prevent end organ damage and/or consumptive coagulopathy [23]. Conservative medical management is the first-line therapy in most cases of PPH and can include uterine massage, uterine packing, transfusion, administration of uterotonic drugs such as oxytocin, and correction of coagulopathy [5]. Etiologies of PPH that necessitate urgent hysterectomy include uterine rupture and uterine inversion [30].

Indications/Contraindications

Image-guided percutaneous embolization should be considered if PPH is caused by uterine atony, uterine tears, or surgical complications from caesarean section, onset of bleeding in the recovery unit, and bleeding following hysterectomy [31]. Studies have also suggested that embolization is a useful adjunct treatment for patients with refractory PPH [32]. Hysterectomy is commonly employed to manage PPH; however, this will lead to infertility and is reserved as a last resort in most cases. If embolization fails, clinicians may consider reattempting it before moving on to hysterectomy [33]. Prophylactic and elective embolization is indicated in cases of placenta accreta known or suspected based on past deliveries or diagnostic imaging [31].

Procedure

There are some variations in the specific details of the procedure depending on provider preference; presented here is a common approach to embolization of the uterine artery.

- This procedure is usually performed under conscious sedation with local anesthetic at the access site [12].
- Using Seldinger technique, common femoral artery access is obtained under palpation or ultrasound guidance into the right common femoral artery [34].
- A catheter is threaded over the wire through the femoral artery into the distal abdominal aorta [30].
- Angiography of the uterine arteries is performed bilaterally to characterize bleeding location and rate prior to embolization [12].
- Threshold for detection of hemorrhage on angiography is contrast medium extravasation at a rate of more than 1–2 mL/min.
- Bleeding may not be visualized if rate is too slow or intermittent or uterine atony is the cause [12].
- Previous studies have visualized extravasation in 42% of cases [35], and empiric embolization is recommended in cases where patients present clinical signs of ongoing hemorrhage [30].
- Many embolization agents can be used including polyvinyl alcohol (PVA) particles, gelatin sponge (Gelfoam), and cyanoacrylate.
- Gelfoam is the preferred embolization agent because vasculature can be recanalized several weeks later, while PVA particle and cyanoacrylate embolization are both more permanent [5, 12].

Outcomes and Complications

The end point for embolization is the absence of contrast medium extravasation on fluoroscopy if it was visualized on previous fluoroscopy [34]. Overall success rates of embolization for PPH range from 71.5 to 88.6% on retrospective reviews of centers performing the procedure and have been reported as 90.7% by literature review [12, 36]. Overall complication rate reported in medical literature varies from 0 to 14.3% [30]. Major complications are rare and include hemorrhage, re-intervention (either re-embolization or alternative management including hysterectomy), internal iliac artery perforation, transient fever, transient buttock or foot ischemia, vaginal or uterine necrosis, and abscess [30, 32, 34].

Placenta Accreta

Definition

Placenta accreta is the abnormal insertion and penetration of placental tissue into the endometrial lining of the uterus [12]. It is divided into three subtypes depending on the degree of penetration of placental tissue: placenta accreta vera (placental penetration into myometrium), placenta increta (deep penetration into myometrium), and placenta percreta (penetration through serosal layer of uterus and possibly surrounding tissues) [37]. This condition may lead to intrapartum and postpartum hemorrhage [12].

Epidemiology and Risk Factors

The incidence rate of placenta accreta is estimated to be approximately 1 per 533 pregnancies, and increases in the incidence rate over the past 20 years are attributed to higher rates of caesarean section [38, 39]. Risk factors for this condition include placenta previa with previous caesarean section or uterine surgery, maternal age >35 years, higher number of births (parity), presence of submucous uterine fibroids, history of smoking, and endometrial defects [12, 40]. Reduction in hemorrhage rates and morbidity during delivery has been shown to occur with early antenatal diagnosis and appropriate plan implementation for delivery [41].

Management

Placenta accreta can be managed conservatively (leaving the placenta partially or completely in situ), surgically via local resection or hysterectomy, or through endovascular procedures [42]. Conservative management has been associated with increased risk of hemorrhage and infection, and risk of hysterectomy was determined to be 58% within 9 months of delivery [42].

Endovascular management of placenta accreta involves pre- and intra-procedural balloon vessel occlusion and in some cases uterine artery embolization both as adjunct therapy with hysterectomy and primary therapy [12]. Recent literature shows that variation exists in the details of the procedure. For example, balloon vessel occlusion can be performed at the level of the internal iliac arteries, the common iliac artery, or the aorta [42, 43].

Pre- and Intra-Balloon Vessel Occlusion Procedure, Outcomes, and Complications

Prophylactic balloon occlusion of internal iliac arteries was reported first by Dubois et al. [44]. The primary goal of balloon vessel occlusion is to minimize bleeding in the pre-, intra-, and postpartum setting as well as increase the probability of retaining the uterus and placenta for future fertility by reducing the need for caesarean hysterectomy (Fig. 16.3).

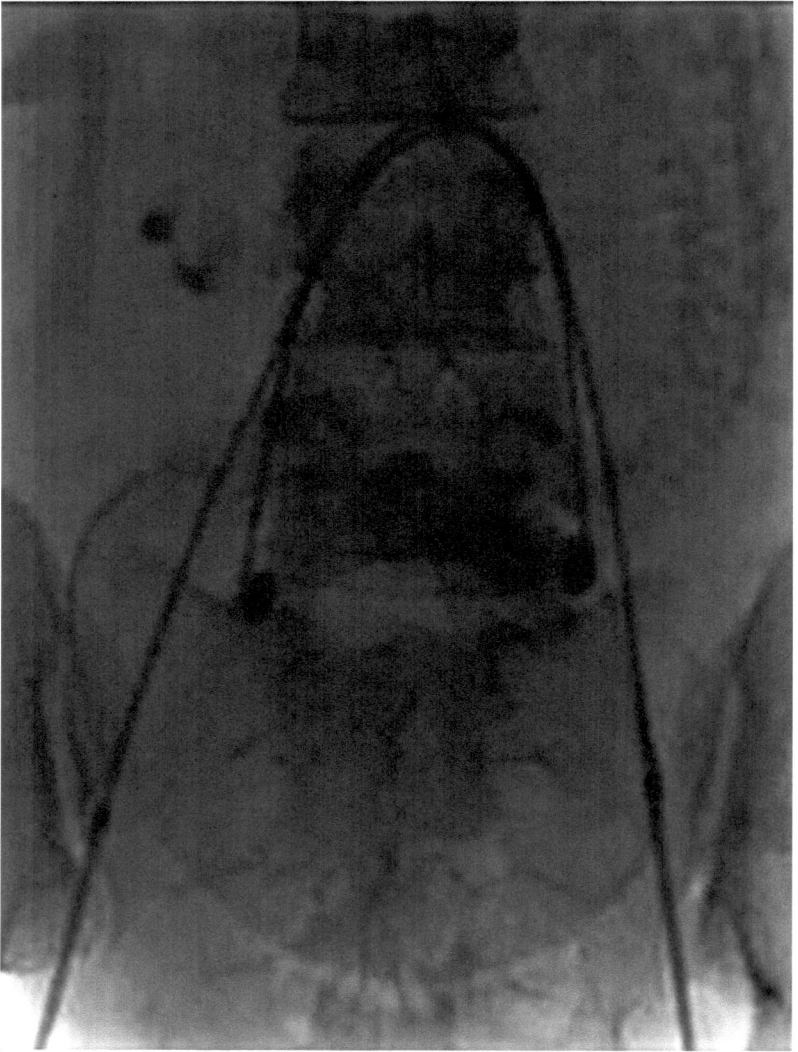

Fig. 16.3 Bilateral internal iliac balloon occlusion for treatment of placenta accreta imaged intraprocedurally on fluoroscopy

Procedure

The common femoral arteries are accessed bilaterally using a Seldinger technique. A balloon catheter is placed into the main trunk of the contralateral internal iliac arteries on each side, with adequate positioning confirmed on angiography during test inflation of the balloon. Therapeutic inflation of the balloon will occur immediately after fetal removal and clamping of the umbilical cord.

Outcomes

The literature on outcomes for this procedure is primarily case reports, retrospective reviews, and case-control studies [45]. Investigated outcomes include amount of blood loss intraoperatively, amount of blood transfused, length of stay in hospital, rate of caesarean hysterectomy, and mortality. Only one study shows reduction in the amount of blood loss and transfusion requirement, while other studies have shown no benefit, and all studies have shown no effect on the length of stay [45]. No mortality has been reported related to this procedure [45].

Complications

The main complications from this procedure are catheter-related complications [45]. The complications are reported primarily in individual case reports and include thromboembolic events leading to acute limb ischemia, vessel pseudoaneurysm, arterial rupture, and stent placement with or without arterial bypass [45].

Uterine Artery Embolization Procedure and Complications

The first use of embolization as primary therapy for placenta accreta was done by Mitty et al. [46]. The technical details of uterine artery embolization for placenta accreta are identical to the procedure for uterine fibroid embolization (Fig. 16.2) [12]. Complications of embolization are like those of uterine fibroid embolization; however, embolization for placenta accreta increases recurrence risk of abnormal placental invasion in future pregnancy [12].

UAE Outcomes

Endovascular therapy is primarily an adjunct treatment along with hysterectomy, local resection, or conservative management of placenta accreta, and the outcome is dependent on the primary therapy method selected [12]. There have been demonstrated cases of pregnancy following embolization as primary therapy for placenta accreta, suggesting that patients considering future pregnancy may benefit from uterine artery embolization over hysterectomy in some cases [12].

Pelvic Congestion Syndrome (PCS)

Overview

Pelvic congestion syndrome is a common cause of chronic (lasting over 6 months) pelvic pain occurring due to pelvic vein congestion. This syndrome may be caused by multiple factors including absence or insufficiency of ovarian vein valves, external compression of vasculature such as in the Nutcracker syndrome and the May–Thurner syndrome, ovarian vessel congestion resulting from retrograde blood flow, acquired inferior vena cava syndrome, or portal hypertension (Fig. 16.4a) [12, 47].

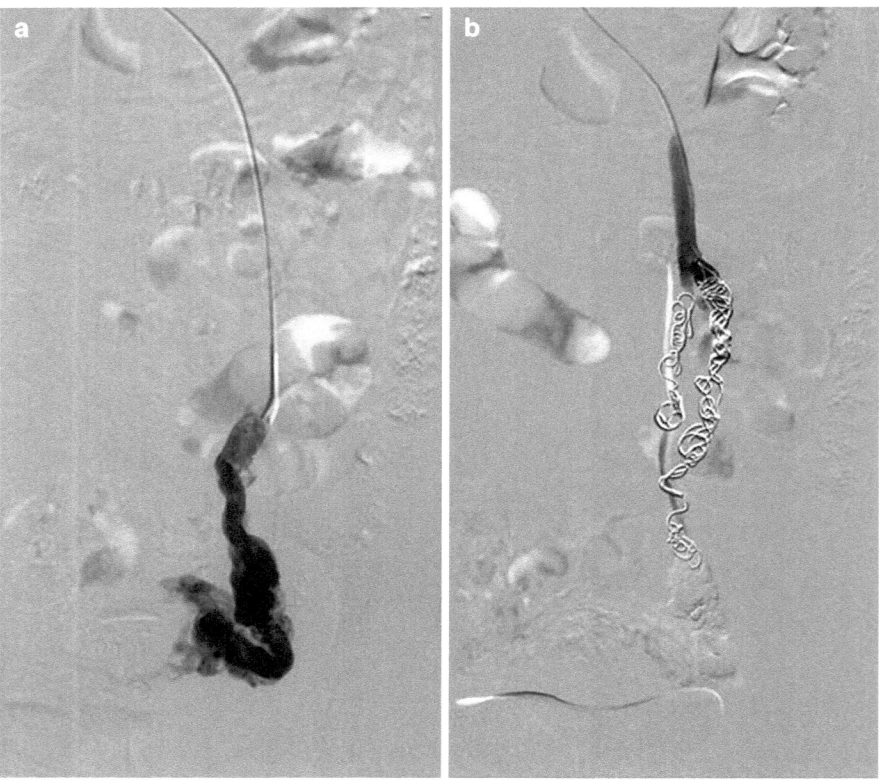

Fig. 16.4 (**a**) Dilated and tortuous left gonadal vein—pelvic congestion syndrome. (**b**) Post-coil embolization of the left-sided pelvic congestion syndrome

Pain symptoms of pelvic congestion syndrome include non-cyclical pain presenting in pregnancy, worsening with subsequent pregnancies, before or during menstruation, after intercourse, exacerbation by fatigue, standing, or any other cause of increased intra-abdominal pressure [12, 47]. Pain can present bilaterally or may alternate sides [47]. Additional symptoms include bladder irritability, increased urinary frequency, and a feeling of fullness in the patient's legs [12].

Epidemiology

Medical literature suggests estimates of 15% prevalence of chronic pelvic pain in women 18–50 years old in the United States and 39% of all women experiencing chronic pelvic pain at some point in their lives [5, 48]. Up to 30% of chronic pelvic pain is associated only with findings characteristic of pelvic congestion syndrome [12]. PCS occurs primarily in premenopausal, multiparous women [49].

Diagnosis and Pre-Procedure Imaging

Although pelvic venous insufficiency may be diagnosed as an incidental finding on abdominopelvic imaging, imaging for patients with pelvic pain is guided by clinical assessment of patient status and clinical suspicion of PCS as well as the exclusion of multiple common causes of pelvic pain [12, 50, 51]. Common causes of pelvic pain that need to be ruled out prior to an exclusive diagnosis of PCS include endometriosis, pelvic inflammatory disease, postoperative adhesions, and uterine fibroids [51].

The imaging modalities that are commonly employed in patients where PCS is suspected are transabdominal and transvaginal duplex ultrasonography, contrast-enhanced CT scan of abdomen and pelvis, or MRI with pelvic venography for diagnostic confirmation [12, 50]. Duplex ultrasound is commonly the preferred diagnostic test, while pelvic venography is the gold standard [47]. The reported cut-off values for ovarian vein diameter differ between imaging techniques. On venography, an ovarian vein diameter of 6 mm and greater is one of the five criteria scored to diagnose PCS [47]. On MRI, ovarian vein incompetence is defined as a measured diameter of more than 8 mm at a point 10 mm from the termination of the vessel [50]. Reflux into venous plexus is graded using Doppler ultrasound or dynamic MR angiography [50]. Laparoscopy is not commonly used for diagnostic purposes of PCS; the pelvic vasculature is poorly visualized as CO_2 insufflation commonly causes venous collapse [47].

Procedure

Catheterization for the procedure is performed using jugular or transfemoral access based on operator preference [52–54]. After appropriate localization and positioning, the primary embolization approach is the placement of endovascular coils in the right and left ovarian veins bilaterally (Fig. 16.4b) [51]. Some interventionalists also perform pelvic vein sclerosis using a mixture of 5% sodium morrhuate and Gelfoam in addition to coil placement for embolization of pelvic veins [54, 55].

Outcomes

The goals of the ovarian vein embolization are technical success characterized by pelvic venous stasis measured by contrast medium flow on venography and clinical success characterized by patient symptom relief on history and examination [51]. Reports in medical literature vary in treatment success from 70 to 100% of patients treated [51]. Pelvic pain recurrence rate has not been studied extensively, but preliminary data shows a recurrence rate of 5–8% [47, 56].

Complications

Complications from this procedure are infrequent, occurring in less than 5% of cases [57]. Complications include thrombophlebitis, spasm and rupture of ovarian vein, and aberrant coil embolization through the IVC into the pulmonary arteries [57].

Inferior Vena Cava (IVC) Filters in Pregnancy

Overview

Venous thromboembolism (VTE) causes substantial mortality in pregnancy [12]. Vitamin K antagonists are teratogenic, and side effects are associated with long-term use of low-molecular-weight heparins [58].

Indications

IVC filters are indicated for pregnant patients with contraindications to medical anticoagulation therapy who have developed VTE during pregnancy [12]. IVC filters should not be placed prophylactically and only provide survival advantage during periods of acute risk for venous thromboembolic disease, with confirmed lower limb DVT or with proximal DVTs prior to labor [12, 58].

Procedure and Equipment

The procedure for IVC filter placement in pregnant women is identical to that of other patients, with the addition of abdominal shielding to minimize radiation dose delivered to the fetus. Additionally, the IVC filter may be placed suprarenally as the infrarenal IVC may be compressed by the growing uterus [59]. A retrievable IVC filter is preferred as placement is acutely based on VTE risk and should be removed when risk decreases [12]. Retrievable IVC filters include Gunther Tulip, Optease, Recovery Nitinol, and Cook Celect [12]. Permanent (Greenfield) IVC filters are not indicated due to high rates of complications including insertion site thrombosis, IVC thrombosis, IVC wall penetration, filter migration, and postphlebitic syndrome [12].

Complications

Complications for IVC filters in pregnancy are identical to those in nonpregnant patients and include delayed filter removal, filter tilt, caval wall perforation, filter damage due to guide wire entanglement, migration of filter, post-thrombotic syndrome, and IVC thrombosis or stenosis [12].

Uterine Arteriovenous Fistula (AVF)

Overview

AVFs are abnormal connections between arteries and veins without a corresponding set of capillaries. They can be congenital or acquired and can occur in any part of the body [12]. Uterine AVFs specifically are abnormal communication between uterine arteries and myometrial veins when acquired or between pelvic arteries and veins when congenital (Fig. 16.5) [60]. Depending on the etiology, location, and other patient factors, AVFs may pose life-threatening hemorrhagic risk to patients [12]. AVFs range from asymptomatic to presenting with severe menorrhagia, and diagnosis can be made using MRI, hysteroscopy, or arteriogram of the area [12, 63]. Symptoms of uterine AVFs include severe menorrhagia, infertility or recurrent pregnancy loss, lower abdominal pain, dyspareunia, asymptomatic pulsatile masses in the pelvis, and anemia secondary to hemorrhage [12, 60].

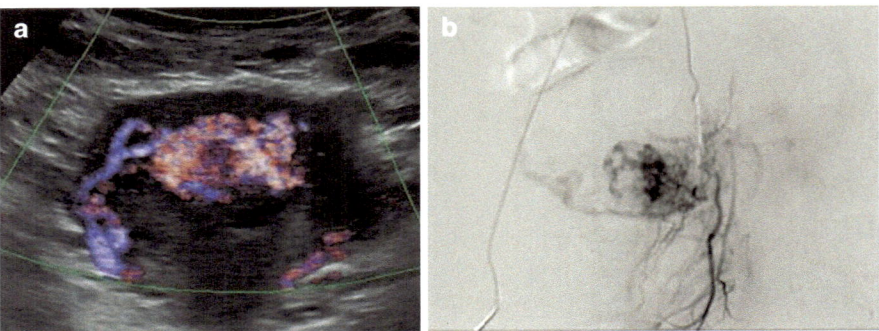

Fig. 16.5 (**a**) Ultrasound image showing uterine arteriovenous malformation (AVM) following D&C. (**b**) Left uterine angiogram confirming uterine AVM

Etiology and Epidemiology

Uterine AVFs are a very rare condition: reports in medical literature suggest they are present in 1–4.5% of patients with pelvic bleeding, while the true incidence is still unknown [60–62]. Acquired AVFs primarily occur in women of reproductive age but have been reported in the literature in patients ranging from 18 to 72 years old [64]. Imaging diagnosis of AVFs is primarily done using color and spectral flow Doppler ultrasonography; however, it can also be completed using CT or MRI. Fluoroscopic angiography is still considered gold standard although currently it is primarily used for cases requiring embolization [60, 61]. A list of the causes of congenital and acquired uterine AVFs is presented in Table 16.1; however, the incidence rate of each etiology is not currently known [12, 60].

Management

The management of AVFs depends on many factors including presentation, severity of symptoms, hemodynamic stability, and patient characteristics including the desire to retain future fertility and age [12, 61]. Acutely, the primary management goal is hemodynamic stabilization and bleeding control using medical measures including uterine packing, 15-methyl-prostaglandin $F_{2\alpha}$, estrogen, progestin, methylergonovine, and danazol [61]. In the past, definitive management for symptomatic AVFs was hysterectomy with possible internal iliac artery ligation following hemodynamic stabilization [12]. In hemodynamically stable patients with low symptomatic burden, observation has been shown to be effective, as over 60% of AVFs diagnosed by ultrasound resolved spontaneously in one study [65]. Transcatheter embolization of AVFs using embolization agents including metallic coils, PVA, Gelfoam, and N-butyl cyanoacrylate has shown to be appropriate both in urgent and non-acute setting [61].

Table 16.1 Causes of AVFs
[12, 60]

Cause	Type
Abnormal development of primitive vasculature	Congenital
Endometrial carcinoma	Acquired
Exposure to diethylstilbestrol	Acquired
Gestational trophoblastic disease	Acquired
Induced abortion	Acquired
Previous uterine surgery (curettage, caesarean section, hysterectomy)	Acquired
Removal of intrauterine contraceptive device	Acquired
Trauma	Acquired

Outcomes

Due to the scarcity of data, the majority of outcome information comes from case series in the literature. Uterine artery embolization has been shown to have a clinical success rate of 93% and a technical success rate of 100% in one study, with long-term success rate of 79 and 90% in two additional studies [66–68]. Successful pregnancies following this embolization procedure have been reported in the literature. An observational study published in 2021 described a period of 3 ± 3 months from embolization to pregnancy [69]. However, more work needs to be done to characterize fertility following this procedure [70].

Complications

Reported complications of transcatheter embolization for uterine AVFs include non-flow-limiting dissection of internal iliac artery, post-embolic pelvic pain, and repeat embolization, while suggested longer-term complications include growth restriction, uterine atony, and uterine rupture [12, 61, 66]. Complication rates in the literature have been very low, averaging less than 4% overall [66].

Fallopian Tube Recanalization

Definitions

- Hysterosalpingogram (HSG): the visualization under fluoroscopy of the shape of the uterine cavity as well as the shape and patency of fallopian tubes through the injection of radio-opaque contrast.

- Selective salpingography (SSG): the use of a radiographic tubal assessment set (RTAS) to image each fallopian tube separately by threading a catheter to the utero-tubal junction [71].
- Falloposcopy: the examination of fallopian tubes using a micro-endoscope.

Overview

Selective tubal catheterization has emerged as a treatment for infertility and subfertility in women diagnosed with proximal fallopian tube obstruction. It is performed by threading a catheter through the uterus and using contrast to image the utero-tubal junction as well as the flow of contrast through the fallopian tubes. If an obstruction is observed, an attempt is made to pass the catheter through the obstruction and reopen the tube. The success rate of this procedure varies depending on the type of imaging guidance used, and it is one of several treatments that can be used to manage infertility and subfertility in women. It can be unilateral or bilateral.

Epidemiology

Tubal-related conditions are associated with 25–30% of female infertility or subfertility worldwide [70]. Of women with tubal-related infertility or subfertility, 10–25% have proximal obstruction which is caused by pelvic inflammatory disease, endometriosis, and tubal spasms among others [72, 73]. One challenge with effectively determining the prevalence of proximal tubal obstruction is the very high rate of false-positive rate of diagnosis on HSG compared to selective salpingography or resected fallopian tubes examined in pathology [71].

Indications/Contraindications

This procedure is indicated in patients with diagnosed proximal tubal obstruction and clinical signs of infertility or subfertility. This procedure particularly benefits patients desiring natural conception in the future [45]. Recanalization of fallopian tubes is best performed in the follicular phase of the menstrual cycle prior to ovulation. Contraindications for this procedure include active pelvic infection, contrast allergy, pelvic malignancy, bilateral tubal disease, and current pregnancy [73].

Procedure

This procedure is performed primarily under selective fluoroscopic guidance, hysteroscopy, ultrasonography, and falloposcopy [72]. Under imaging guidance, the patency of the fallopian tubes is assessed by visualizing contrast flow through each fallopian tube [72]. A catheter is threaded through the obstructed region of the fallopian tube until patency is achieved on imaging [72].

Intra-Procedural Imaging Guidance and Procedure Success

One of the main challenges with this procedure is variability in uterine position, which may decrease the success rate of tubal canalization [5]. Procedure success may also be affected by uterine malformations and the presence of polyps or uterine fibroids [5]. The success rate for pregnancy and live birth following recanalization was shown to be higher in unilateral proximal tubal obstruction (Table 16.2) [72].

Complications

The main described complications of this procedure are cramping and vaginal bleeding, both of which are mild and usually self-limiting [5]. More serious complications include tubal perforation, adnexal infection, and future ectopic pregnancy [5]. Depending on the type of imaging guidance used, there are risks associated with ovarian radiation exposure if selective salpingography is used [5]. If the fallopian tubes become re-occluded, the recanalization procedure can be repeated [72].

Table 16.2 Characterizing the effectiveness of fallopian tube recanalization using different types of imaging guidance [72, 73]

Type of imaging guidance	Mean rate of successful cannulation (%) (range)	Mean pregnancy rate reported (%) (range)	Mean live birth rate reported (%) (range)
Selective salpingography	68% (31–100%)	34% (22–55%)	32.3% (32–36%)
Laparoscopy	61.5% (37–88%)	35% (23.5–43%)	16.7% (14.8–23.5%)
Ultrasonography	84% (no range)	16% (no range)	NR
Falloposcopy	81.6% (no range)	29.9% (no range)	NR

Acknowledgment We would like to thank Dr. Lazar Milovanovic for his contributions to this chapter (information given on first page of chapter).

References

1. Ravina JH, Herbreteau D, Ciraru-Vigneron N, et al. Arterial embolization to treat uterine myomata. Lancet. 1995;46(8976):671–2.
2. Christman GM. Uterine leiomyomas. Clinical reproductive medicine and surgery. New York: Springer; 2017.
3. Buttram VC Jr, Reiter RC. Uterine leiomyomata: etiology, symptomatology, and management. Fertil Steril. 1981;36(4):433–45.
4. Baird DD, Dunson DB, Hill MC, Cousins D, Schectman JM. High cumulative incidence of uterine leiomyoma in black and white women: ultrasound evidence. Am J Obstet Gynecol. 2003;188:100–7.
5. Lopera J, Suri R, Kroma GM, Garza-Berlanga A, Thomas J. Role of interventional procedures in obstetrics/gynecology. Radiol Clin North Am. 2013;51:1049–66.
6. Stovall DW, Parrish SB, Van Voorhis BJ, Hahn SJ, Sparks AE, Syrop CH. Uterine leiomyomas reduce the efficacy of assisted reproduction cycles: results of a matched follow-up study. Hum Reprod. 1998;13(1):192–7.
7. Rein MS, Barbieri RL, Friedman AJ. Progesterone: a critical role in the pathogenesis of uterine myomas. Am J Obstet Gynecol. 1995;172(1 pt 1):14–8.
8. Stokes LS, Wallace MJ, Godwin RB, Kundu S, Cardella JF. Quality improvement guidelines for uterine artery embolization for symptomatic leiomyomas. J Vasc Interv Radiol. 2010;21:1153–63.
9. Hooks-Anderson D. Uterine fibroid. Salem Press encyclopedia of health. Hackensack: Salem Press; 2019.
10. Abbara S, Nikolic B, Pelage JP, Banovac F, Spies JB. Frequency and extent of uterine perfusion via ovarian arteries observed during uterine artery embolization for leiomyomas. Am J Roentgenol. 2007;188:1558.
11. Burn PR, McCall JM, Chinn RJ, Vashisht A, Smith JR, Healy JC. Uterine fibroleiomyoma: MR imaging appearance before and after embolization of uterine arteries. Radiology. 2000;214:729–34.
12. Ganeshan A, Nazir SA, Hon LQ, et al. The role of interventional radiology in obstetric and gynaecology practice. Eur J Radiol. 2010;73:404–11.
13. Bratby MJ, Ramachandran N, Sheppard N, Kyriou J, Munneke GM, Belli AM. Prospective study of elective bilateral versus unilateral femoral arterial puncture for uterine artery embolization. Cardiovasc Intervent Radiol. 2007;30:1139–43.
14. Schirf BE, Vogelzang RL, Christman HB. Complications of uterine fibroid embolization. Semin Intervent Radiol. 2006;23(2):143–9.
15. Martin J, Bhanot K, Athreya S. Complications and reinterventions in uterine artery embolization for symptomatic uterine fibroids: a literature review and meta analysis. Cardiovasc Intervent Radiol. 2013;36:395–402.
16. SOGC Clinical Practice Guidelines. Uterine fibroid embolization (UFE). Int J Gynaecol Obstet. 2005;89(3):305–18.
17. Stewart JK. Uterine artery embolization for uterine fibroids: a closer look at misperceptions and challenges. Tech Vasc Interv Radiol. 2021;24(1):100725. https://doi.org/10.1016/j.tvir.2021.100725.
18. Manyonda IT, Bratby M, Horst JS, Banu N, Gorti M, Belli AM. Uterine artery embolization versus myomectomy: impact on quality of life—results of the FUME (Fibroids of the Uterus:

Myomectomy versus Embolization) Trial. Cardiovasc Intervent Radiol. 2012;35(3):530–6. https://doi.org/10.1007/s00270-011-0228-5.

19. Lee MS, Kim MD, Lee M, Won JY, Park SI, Lee DY, Lee KH. Contrast-enhanced MR angiography of uterine arteries for the prediction of ovarian artery embolization in 349 patients. J Vasc Interv Radiol. 2012;23(9):1174–9.

20. Korff RA, Warhit M, Jagust MB, Golowa YS, Cynamon J. The role of non-contrast cone beam CT in identifying incomplete treatment during uterine artery embolization. J Vasc Interv Radiol. 2019;30(5):679–86.

21. Davis MR, Soliman AM, Castelli-Haley J, Snabes MC, Surrey ES. Reintervention rates after myomectomy, endometrial ablation, and uterine artery embolization for patients with uterine fibroids. J Womens Health. 2018;27(10):1204–14.

22. Cope AG, Young RJ, Stewart EA. Non-extirpative treatments for uterine myomas: measuring success. J Minim Invasive Gynecol. 2021;28(3):442–52. https://doi.org/10.1016/j.jmig.2020.08.016.

23. Pacagnella RC, Souza JP, Durocher J, et al. A systematic review of the relationship between blood loss and clinical signs. PLoS One. 2013;8(3):e57594. https://doi.org/10.1371/journal.pone.0057594.

24. Feinberg BB, Resnik E, Hurt WG, Bump RC, Kubota R, Cho SR. Angiographic embolization in the management of late postpartum haemorrhage. J Reprod Med. 1987;32(12):921–31.

25. Jouppila P. Postpartum haemorrhage. Curr Opin Obstet Gynecol. 1995;7(6):446–50.

26. Ledee N, Ville Y, Musset D, Mercier F, Frydman R, Fernandez H. Management in intractable obstetric haemorrhage: an audit study on 61 cases. Eur J Obstet Gynecol Reprod Biol. 2001;94(2):189–96.

27. Chang J, Elam-Evans LD, Berg CJ, et al. Pregnancy-related mortality surveillance—United States, 1991–1999. MMWR Surveill Summ. 2003;52(SS02):1–8.

28. Mousa HA, Alfirevic Z. Treatment for primary postpartum haemorrhage. Cochrane Database Syst Rev. 2007;1(1):CD003249. https://doi.org/10.1002/14651858.CD003249.pub2.

29. Evensen A, Anderson JM, Fontaine P. Postpartum hemorrhage: prevention and treatment. Am Fam Physician. 2017;95(7):442–9.

30. Josephs SC. Obstetric and gynecologic emergencies: a review of indications and interventional techniques. Semin Intervent Radiol. 2008;25(4):337–46.

31. Royal College of Obstetricians and Gynecologists (RCOG). The role of emergency and elective interventional radiology in postpartum haemorrhage. 2007. https://www.rcog.org.uk/guidance/browse-all-guidance/good-practice-papers/the-role-of-emergency-and-elective-interventional-radiology-in-postpartum-haemorrhage-good-practice-no-6/.

32. Martin J, Abraham T. Uterine artery embolization for post-partum hemorrhage. McMaster Univ Med J. 2014;11(1):21–6.

33. Lee HY, Shin JH, Kim J, Yoon HK, Ko GY, Won HS, et al. Primary postpartum hemorrhage: outcome of pelvic arterial embolization in 251 patients at a single institution. Radiology. 2012;264(3):903–9.

34. Gipson MG, Smith MT. Endovascular therapies for primary postpartum hemorrhage: techniques and outcomes. Semin Intervent Radiol. 2013;30:333–9.

35. Boulleret C, Chahid T, Gallot D, Mofid R, Tran HD, Ravel A, et al. Hypogastric arterial selective and superselective embolization for severe postpartum hemorrhage: a retrospective review of 36 cases. Cardiovasc Intervent Radiol. 2004;27:344–8.

36. Doumouchtsis SK, Papageorghiou AT, Arulkumaran S. Systematic review of conservative management of postpartum haemorrhage; what to do when medical treatment fails. Obstet Gynecol Surv. 2007;62:540–7.

37. Breen JL, Nuebecker R, Gregori CA, Franklin JE Jr. Placenta accreta, increta, and percreta: survey of 40 cases. Obstet Gynecol. 1977;49:43–7.

38. Wu S, Kocherginsky M, Hibbard JU. Abnormal placentation: twenty-year analysis. Am J Obstet Gynecol. 2005;192(5):515–20.

39. Ballas J, Hull AD, Saenz C, et al. Preoperative intravascular balloon catheters and surgical outcomes in pregnancies complicated by placenta accreta: a management paradox. Am J Obstet Gynecol. 2012;207(3):e1–5.
40. Guy GP, Peisner DB, Timor-Trisch IE. Ultrasonographic evaluation of uteroplacental blood flow patterns of abnormally located and adherent placentas. Am J Obstet Gynecol. 1990;163(3):723–7.
41. Hong TM, Tseng HS, Lee RC, Wang JH, Chang CY. Uterine artery embolization: an effective treatment for intractable obstetric haemorrhage. Clin Radiol. 2004;59(1):96–101.
42. Clausen C, Lonn L, Langhoff-Roos J. Management of placenta percreta: a review of published cases. Acta Obstet Gynecol Scand. 2013;93:138–43.
43. Shrivastava VK, Ramos GA, Nageotte MP. Role of interventional radiology in the management of abnormal placentation. In: Placenta accreta syndrome. 1st ed. New York: CRC; 2017. p. 105–12.
44. Dilauro MD, Dason S, Athreya S. Prophylactic balloon occlusion of internal iliac arteries in women with placenta accreta: literature review and analysis. Clin Radiol. 2012;67(6):515–20.
45. Tanaka Y, Tajima H. Falloposcopic tuboplasty as an option for tubal infertility: an alternative to in vitro fertilization. Fertil Steril. 2011;95(1):441–3.
46. Mitty HA, Sterling KM, Alvarez M, Gendler R. Obstetric haemorrhage: prophylactic and emergency arterial catheterization and embolotherapy. Radiology. 1993;188(1):183–7.
47. Desai N, Dassel M. Pelvic pain arising from pelvic congestion syndrome. In: Hibner M, editor. Management of chronic pelvic pain: a practical manual. Cambridge: Cambridge University Press; 2021. p. 112–9. https://doi.org/10.1017/9781108877084.011.
48. Mathias SD, Kuppermann M, Liberman RF, Lipschutz RC, Steege JF. Chronic pelvic pain: prevalence, health-related quality of life, and economic correlates. Obstet Gynecol. 1996;87(3):321–7.
49. Beard RW, Pearce S, Highman JH, Reginald PW. Diagnosis of pelvic varicosities in women with chronic pelvic pain. Lancet. 1984;324(8409):946–9.
50. Leiber LM, Thouveny F, Bouvier A, et al. MRI and venographic aspects of pelvic venous insufficiency. Diagn Interv Imaging. 2014;94:1091–102. https://doi.org/10.1016/j.diii.2014.01.012.
51. Durham JD, Machlan L. Pelvic congestion syndrome. Semin Intervent Radiol. 2013;30(4):372–80.
52. Hocquelet A, Le Bras Y, Balian E, Bouzgarrou M, Myer M, Rigou G, et al. Evaluation of the efficacy of endovascular treatment of pelvic congestion syndrome. Diagn Interv Imaging. 2014;95:301–6.
53. Nasser F, Cavalcante RN, Affonso BB, Messina ML, Carnevale FC, de Gregorio MA. Safety, efficacy, and prognostic factors in endovascular treatment of pelvic congestion syndrome. Int J Gynaecol Obstet. 2014;125:65–8.
54. Ignacio EA, Dua R IV, Sarin S, et al. Pelvic congestion syndrome: diagnosis and treatment. Semin Intervent Radiol. 2008;25(4):361–8.
55. Venbrux AC, Chang AH, Kim HS, et al. Pelvic congestion syndrome (pelvic venous incompetence): impact of ovarian and internal iliac vein embolotherapy on menstrual cycle and chronic pelvic pain. J Vasc Interv Radiol. 2002;13(2 pt 1):171–8.
56. Kim HS, Malhotra AD, Rowe PC, Lee JM, Venbrux AC. Embolotherapy for pelvic congestion syndrome: long-term results. J Vasc Interv Radiol. 2006;17(2pt. 1):289–97.
57. Rane N, Leyon JJ, Littlehales T, Ganeshan A, Crowe P, Uberoi R. Pelvic congestion syndrome. Curr Probl Diagn Radiol. 2013;42(4):135–40.
58. Harvey JJ, Hopkins J, McCafferty IJ, Jones RG. Inferior vena cava filters: what radiologists need to know. Clin Radiol. 2013;68(7):721–32.
59. Crosby DA, Ryan K, McEniff N, Dicker P, Regan C, Lynch C, et al. Retrievable inferior vena cava filters in pregnancy: risk versus benefit? Eur J Obstet Gynecol Reprod Biol. 2018;222:25–30.
60. Cura M, Martinez N, Cura A, Dalsaso TJ, Elmerhi F. Arteriovenous malformations of the uterus. Acta Radiol. 2009;50(7):823–9.

61. Grivell RM, Reid KM, Mellor A. Uterine arteriovenous malformations: a review of the current literature. Obstet Gynecol Surv. 2005;60(11):761–7.
62. Vijayakumar A, Srinivas A, Chandrashekar BM, Vijayakumar A. Uterine vascular lesions. Rev Obstet Gynecol. 2013;6(2):69–79.
63. O'Brien P, Neyastani A, Buckley AR, Chang SD, Legiehn GM. Uterine arteriovenous malformations: from diagnosis to treatment. J Ultrasound Med. 2006;25:1387–92.
64. Arora R, Achla B, Pinkee S, Purba G, Bharti M. Arteriovenous malformations of the uterus. N Z Med J. 2004;117(1206):U1182.
65. Timmerman D, Wauters J, Van Calenbergh S, Van Schoubroeck D, Maleux G, Van Den Bosch T, et al. Color Doppler imaging is a useful tool for the diagnosis and management of uterine vascular malformations. Ultrasound Obstet Gynecol. 2003;21:570–7.
66. Ghai S, Rajan DK, Asch MR, Muradali D, Simons ME, TerBrugge KG. Efficacy of embolization in traumatic uterine vascular malformations. J Vasc Interv Radiol. 2003;14(11):1401–8.
67. Yang JJ, Xiang Y, Wan XR, Yang XY. Diagnosis and management of uterine arteriovenous fistulas with massive vaginal bleeding. Int J Gynecol Obstet. 2005;89(2):114–9.
68. Kwon JH, Kim GS. Obstetric iatrogenic arterial injuries of the uterus: diagnosis with US and treatment with transcatheter arterial embolization. Radiographics. 2002;22(1):35–46.
69. Gilbert A, Thubert T, Dochez V, Riteau AS, Ducloyer M, Ragot P, et al. Angiographic findings and outcomes after embolization of patients with suspected postabortion uterine arteriovenous fistula. J Gynecol Obstet Hum Reprod. 2021;50(7):102033. https://doi.org/10.1016/j.jogoh.2020.102033.
70. Serafini P, Batzofin J. Diagnosis of female infertility. A comprehensive approach. J Reprod Med. 1989;34(1):29–40.
71. Corbellis L, Argano F, Castaldi MA, Acone G, Mele D, Signoriello G, et al. Selective salpingography: preliminary experience of an office operative option for proximal tubal recanalization. Eur J Obstet Gynecol Reprod Biol. 2012;163(1):62–6.
72. Honore GM, Holden AE, Schenken RS. Pathophysiology and management of proximal tubal blockage. Fertil Steril. 1999;71(5):785–95.
73. Hou HY, Chen YQ, Li TC, Hu CX, Chen X, Yang ZH. Outcome of laparoscopy-guided hysteroscopic tubal catheterization for infertility due to proximal tubal obstruction. J Minim Invasive Gynecol. 2014;21(2):272–8.

Chapter 17
Musculoskeletal Interventions

Ibrahim Mohammad Nadeem and Prasaanthan Gopee-Ramanan

Percutaneous Image-Guided Musculoskeletal Biopsy

Background

Bone and soft tissue tumors are a largely heterogeneous group of tumors and often require histopathological studies to establish a definitive diagnosis. In such cases, percutaneous image-guided musculoskeletal biopsy (PMSB) has become a routine procedure. When compared to open biopsy, PMSB has demonstrated lower complication rate with negligible rate of clinically significant complications [1]. PMSB is also better tolerated and less painful and can lead to a definitive diagnosis sooner [1].

Indications and Contraindications

Indications:

• Confirmation or exclusion of a primary or metastatic bone or soft tissue tumor.
• Confirmation or exclusion of infection of the musculoskeletal system.

Contraindications:

• Confidently diagnosed benign lesion with noninvasive imaging modalities.
• Cases where biopsy will not change therapeutic outcome.

I. M. Nadeem (✉) · P. Gopee-Ramanan
Department of Radiology, Faculty of Health Sciences, McMaster University,
Hamilton, ON, Canada
e-mail: ibrahim.nadeem@medportal.ca; prasa.gopee@medportal.ca

© The Author(s), under exclusive license to Springer Nature   193
Switzerland AG 2022
S. Athreya, M. Albahhar (eds.), *Demystifying Interventional Radiology*,
https://doi.org/10.1007/978-3-031-12023-7_17

- Inaccessible or poorly visualized lesion.
- Uncorrected coagulopathy.

Preparation for Biopsy

- Multidisciplinary team should be included in management of the biopsy and consist of an MSK or interventional radiologist, orthopedic sarcoma surgeon, and pathologist.
- Pre-procedural imaging. MRI is the preferred imaging modality for soft tissue tumor and sarcoma evaluation and local staging. Bone lesions are better evaluated with CT.

Procedure

PMSB, like other interventional procedures, is usually performed with either single or dual imaging technique, ultrasound and/or CT, each with its advantages and drawbacks. Most subcutaneous soft tissue masses and soft tissue lesions in the extremities can be biopsied under ultrasound guidance. Generally, a CT scan is performed to localize the lesion precisely and to identify the entry point and pathway while avoiding neurovascular structures. Under sterile conditions and local anesthesia, using a 22-guage needle, the skin, subcutaneous layers, and other structures along the planned pathway are infiltrated with 1% lidocaine anesthetic. The position of the 22-guage needle is confirmed with fluoroscopy and/or CT. Once placement is confirmed, a coaxial biopsy needle is used to obtain samples for histopathological analysis. The apparatus is removed, and direct pressure is applied to the needle entry site until hemostasis is achieved.

Post-Procedural Care

- Monitoring for signs of bleeding.
- Pain management with NSAIDS, paracetamol, or opioids if needed.

Complications

- Hematoma.
- Neural and vascular injuries.
- Fractures.
- Septic osteitis, especially if sterility of the procedure was compromised.
- Reflex sympathetic dystrophy.

Facet Joint Injection

Clinical Background

Focal lower back pain is seen in spinal facet arthropathy; usually this is seen by MSK or interventional radiologists in the context of chronic back pain. Long-standing pain is often coupled with limited range of spinal motion, and pain on paraspinal palpation often helps localize the affected joint(s). Magnetic resonance imaging (MRI) or CT scan of the lower back can be useful for identification after a prolonged period of conservative management with nonsteroidal anti-inflammatory medications (NSAIDs) and prior to procedure [2].

Indications and Contraindications

Indications:

- Pain documented or suspected to be related to facet joint disease.

  Contraindications:

- Active infections are relative contraindications.
- Coagulopathy.

Imaging Required

Pre-procedural plain radiographs, computed tomography (CT), or MRI is advisable to help elucidate anatomy for procedural planning as well as to detect tumors, infections, fractures, or spinal abnormalities.

Pre-Procedure

- Chart review is performed and informed consent obtained.
- The patient is positioned prone on the fluoroscopy table, skin superficial to the facet joints of interest is thoroughly cleansed with chlorhexidine or iodine solution, and sterile draping is placed to designate the sterile field.

Procedure

The fluoroscopy tube is aligned parallel to vertebral disks of interest and the end plates; the tube is obliqued as much as needed to visualize the facet joints of interest. A temporary mark is made on the skin and local anesthesia is achieved using 1%

lidocaine. A 25-gauge spinal needle is inserted and advanced into the facet joint under fluoroscopy; entry is confirmed usually by sensation at the fingertips. Once placement is confirmed by contrast media injection under fluoroscopy, a short Luer-Lock extension tube is attached to the spinal needle hub to inject the steroid mixture, usually 80-mg methylprednisolone acetate in 1 mL together with 1–2 mL of bupivacaine 0.25–0.5% [3]. Sometimes, there is a difficult targeting of or entry into the facet joint due to significant osteophytosis. If intra-articular injection is not possible, a periarticular injection is an appropriate alternative.

Post-Procedure

Lower back pain tends to resolve almost immediately (due to the long-acting anesthetic), thereby confirming the diagnosis and acting as therapy [3]. Variability in how long the steroid's therapeutic effect lasts varies from a few months to 1–2 years [3].

Complications

• Bleeding and infection are rare complications [3].

Percutaneous Vertebral Augmentation

Generally, osteoporosis and malignancy can cause collapse of vertebral bodies resulting in significant pain. If the patient has been unable to receive or has been unsuccessful at responding to medical therapy (i.e., analgesia and pain management), this serves as an indication for percutaneous augmentation of vertebral height (i.e., *vertebroplasty and kyphoplasty*). Percutaneous vertebroplasty is a widely used safe and effective therapeutic option and entails instillation of bone cement (composition) under fluoroscopy [4].

Pre-Procedure

• Contraindications include adequate relief of pain by medical therapy, active local or systemic infection, uncorrectable coagulopathy, and allergy to bone cement products [5].
• Patients are first worked up with history, physical examination, and blood work assessing coagulation status.
• Antiplatelet and anticoagulant therapies are to be held in the week preceding treatment unless otherwise contraindicated.

- MRI is most preferred, namely, the short inversion time inversion recovery (STIR) sequence to identify the acuity of lesions causing vertebral collapse and subsequent symptoms. If an MRI is contraindicated, a nuclear medicine bone scan is acceptable [4].
- Prior to the procedure, a neurological exam should be performed to establish a baseline of neurological status. The procedure involves injection of bone cement, most commonly polymethyl methacrylate (PMMA), into the vertebral body under fluoroscopic guidance (see Fig. 17.1).

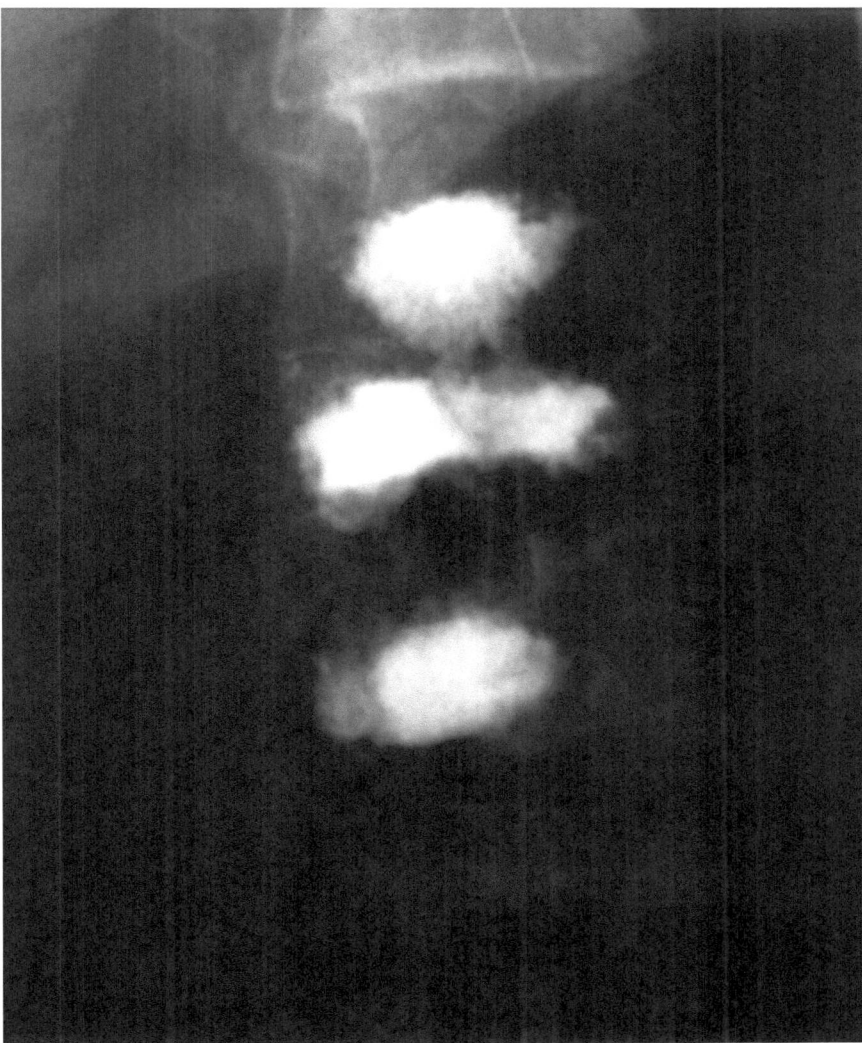

Fig. 17.1 Post-vertebroplasty fluoroscopic image depicting bone cement within lumbar vertebral bodies

Post-Procedure

- Post-procedural care involves application of pressure over the injection site to achieve hemostasis.
- The patient is then kept in a supine position for at least 2 h, after which a neurological exam is repeated.
- Complications include infection, bleeding, transient radiculopathy, cement leak into the spinal canal, and chemical pulmonary embolism [4].

Acknowledgment We would like to thank Dr. Prasaanthan Gopee-Ramanan for his contributions to this chapter (information given on first page of chapter).

References

1. Vasilevska Nikodinovska V, Ivanoski S, Samardziski M, Janevska V. Percutaneous imaging-guided versus open musculoskeletal biopsy: concepts and controversies. Semin Musculoskelet Radiol. 2020;24(6):667–75. https://doi.org/10.1055/s-0040-1717113.
2. Luo QZ, Lin L, Gong Z, et al. Positive association of major histocompatibility complex class I chain-related gene a polymorphism with leukemia susceptibility in the people of Han nationality of Southern China. Tissue Antigens. 2011;78(3):178–84.
3. Stone JA, Bartynski WS. Treatment of facet and sacroiliac joint arthropathy: steroid injections and radiofrequency ablation. Tech Vasc Interv Radiol. 2009;12(1):22–32.
4. Jay B, Ahn SH. Vertebroplasty. Semin Intervent Radiol. 2013;30(3):297–306.
5. Nieuwenhuijse MJ, van Erkel AR, Dijkstra PD. Percutaneous vertebroplasty in very severe osteoporotic vertebral compression fractures: feasible and beneficial. J Vasc Interv Radiol. 2011;22(7):1017–23.

Chapter 18
Interventional Oncology

Lazar Milovanovic and Ashis Bagchee-Clark

Interventional Oncology Procedures

Procedures can be categorized into procedures with diagnostic intent and procedures with therapeutic intent. Diagnostic procedures include fine needle aspiration, core needle biopsy, and vacuum-assisted biopsy; all three are performed with the aim of collecting tissue for histopathology. These procedures are discussed in greater detail in Chap. 7: Biopsy and Drainage. This section will focus on the therapeutic procedures of interventional oncology, which can be used as primary treatment options for patients, but are more frequently used in combination with conventional therapies to augment treatment and improve outcomes [1].

Therapeutic interventional oncology procedures can be further categorized into ablation and embolization procedures. Ablation procedures directly target and destroy neoplastic cells, while embolization procedures do so in an indirect fashion [2]. Both techniques employ image guidance, allowing treatment to be delivered in a minimally invasive fashion through percutaneous techniques.

The different image-guided ablation and embolization techniques are described in Table 18.1. The different conditions these techniques treat, their indications for treatment, and treatment outcomes are outlined in Table 18.2. Table 18.3 contains a summary of the tiers of interventional oncology procedures and examples of procedures performed by interventional oncologists at each step of the treatment process.

L. Milovanovic · A. Bagchee-Clark (✉)
Michael G. DeGroote School of Medicine, McMaster University, Hamilton, ON, Canada
e-mail: lazar.milovanovic@medportal.ca; ashis.bagcheeclark@medportal.ca

Table 18.1 Interventional oncology procedures [2]

Procedure type	Method of action that promotes cell death
Ablation	
Chemical	Injection of chemical substances into the tumor
Radiofrequency	Tissue heating due to frictional energy
Irreversible electroporation	Disrupting cell membrane electric potential gradient
Cryoablation	Intracellular freezing and electrochemical gradient disruption
Microwave	Tissue heating due to electromagnetic energy
High-intensity focused ultrasound	Tissue heating and coagulation due to ultrasonic waves
Embolization	
Transarterial embolization	Infusion of embolic material to occlude an artery feeding the tumor
Intra-arterial chemotherapy	Infusion of chemotherapeutic agents into an artery feeding the tumor
Transarterial chemoembolization (TACE)	Infusion of chemotherapeutic agents then infusion of embolic material into an artery feeding the tumor
Transarterial radioembolization (TARE)	Infusion of radioisotope-loaded microspheres followed by injection of embolic material into an artery feeding the tumor

Table 18.2 Interventional oncology procedures [1]

Procedure	Condition treated	Indication	Outcomes
Intra-arterial therapy (TACE, DEB TACE, bland embolization)	Hepatocellular carcinoma (HCC)	• Patients awaiting transplantation with low MELD scores • Salvage therapy for nonsurgical candidates	• Increased 1, 3, and 5 years of survival Over supportive therapy [6]
Percutaneous ablation (RFA, cryoablation, MWA, IRE)	Liver, lung, and kidney tumors	• Primary therapy in nonsurgical candidates with localized disease to the lung, liver, or kidney • Pain palliation for painful skeletal metastases refractory to alternative treatment	• Depends on specific treatment, RFA most established • Risk factors for survival in HCC include size of dominant lesion, CEA level [1]
Adjuvant treatment Portal vein embolization	Hepatic surgery candidates	• Augmentation of size of future liver remnant prior to surgery	Palliative
Adjuvant treatment Percutaneous biliary drainage	Hepatobiliary or pancreatic cancer	• Biliary drainage due to symptoms of biliary obstruction secondary to invasion and/or compression of ducts by tumor	Palliative

TACE transarterial chemoembolization, *DEB TACE* drug-eluting bead transarterial chemoembolization, *RFA* radiofrequency ablation, *MWA* microwave ablation, *IRE* irreversible electroporation, *MELD* model for end-stage liver disease

Table 18.3 Tiers of interventional oncology

Goal of intervention	Examples of IO procedures performed by IRs
Tissue diagnosis	CT-, US-, or fluoroscopy-guided biopsy
Symptomatic treatment	Nephrostomy for obstructive bladder cancer
Palliation	Embolization for bleeding renal/bladder cancer SVC stenting for SVCO. Tracheal, esophageal, gastroduodenal and colonic stenting. Feeding GI tubes Pain relief
Supplemental care	Port-a-cath placement
Bridge to surgery/chemotherapy	TACE for hepatic tumors, colonic stenting
Therapeutic	Tumor ablation

IO interventional oncology, *CT* computed tomography, *US* ultrasound, *SVC* superior vena cava, *SVCO* superior vena cava obstruction, *GI* gastrointestinal, *TACE* transcatheter arterial chemoembolization

Role of Imaging in Interventional Oncology

Imaging in interventional oncology is used for pre-procedural treatment planning, intraprocedural targeting and monitoring, and post-procedural monitoring. Imaging for interventional oncology prioritizes real-time imaging with decreased scan time and reduced radiation dose over diagnostic highest-quality imaging [3]. During pre-procedural treatment planning, the highest-quality imaging is desired and can involve both anatomic (computed tomography [CT], magnetic resonance imaging [MRI]) and physiologic (single-photon emission computed tomography [SPECT], positron emission tomography [PET]) imaging. Pre-procedure imaging needs to assess whether the procedure is medically indicated, whether the procedure is technically feasible, and how to best approach the target for therapy including anatomic variants and relevant nearby structures.

Current approaches for intraprocedural targeting include the use of CT, fluoroscopy, MRI, and ultrasound as two-dimensional planar imaging for localization during treatment. Most of the currently available angio-interventional equipment offers 3D imaging and targeting of the lesions for various interventions.

For intraprocedural monitoring, an important challenge in interventional oncology is to assess the adequacy of treatment using parameters known to change as the procedure is completed. Examples of intraprocedural indicators include blood flow assessment for post-embolization evaluation, contrast-agent uptake, and magnetic resonance perfusion among others.

After the procedure is completed, imaging is used periodically to evaluate the effectiveness of the treatment and determine complications, recurrence, or other adverse results. Post-procedural imaging focuses on tissue enhancement and nodular growth on serial imaging.

Tumor Board/Multidisciplinary Rounds

Treating cancer is rarely unimodal: given the many different cancer treatments and their different mechanisms of action destroying neoplastic cells, greatest healthcare outcomes are often observed when oncologists and other physicians across a range of disciplines are involved in the care of a patient. Other healthcare professionals also vital in achieving best possible patient outcomes include nurses, pathologists, genetic counselors, social workers, and physical and occupational therapists.

Consequently, multidisciplinary rounds are an important part of the patient-centered care model for managing cancer; they provide a place for diagnostic and treatment clarification between radiologists, pathologists, medical oncologists, surgeons, and radiation oncologists. Radiologists currently play a crucial role in the diagnosis and characterization of malignancy, with interventional radiologists often conducting minimally invasive tissue biopsies to collect tissue samples for pathological analysis, while diagnostic radiologists assess imaging scans in order to characterize end-stage cancer patients.

Current Trends in Interventional Oncology

Interventional oncology is an exciting and growing modality within the field of oncology [4–7]. Interventional oncology has transformed the landscape of cancer care; for example, in the treatment of hepatocellular carcinoma, it allows for chemotherapy to be preferentially delivered to areas of greater amount of cancerous tissue [8, 9]. The emergence of increasing evidence for embolization, chemoembolization, and ablative therapy for the treatment of malignant lesions has led to further focused research within many different areas of interventional oncology and the utilization of novel interventional radiology devices and procedures for primary, adjuvant, supportive, and palliative treatment in oncology practices. Drug-eluting beads are one example: many newer microspheres used for embolization possess an electrical charge that allows a specific chemotherapeutic agent, such as irinotecan, to be loaded and thus delivered in a localized fashion; however, there remains many effective chemotherapeutic agents which cannot currently be loaded on existing microspheres [10]. There is also the potential for a synergistic effect between interventional oncology and immunotherapy, another expanding cancer care modality, and this is a current area of research [11].

Clinical trials recently completed and currently underway focus on characterizing the specific role of interventional oncology procedures and their survival rates, morbidity, and mortality relative to current standard therapies [4–7]. Interventional oncology is now often considered the fourth pillar of cancer care, alongside surgery, radiation oncology and medical oncology [12] and can function as primary therapy or in conjunction with other therapies [13].

References

1. Smith KA, Kim HS. Interventional radiology and image-guided medicine: interventional oncology. Semin Oncol. 2011;38(1):151–62.
2. Hickey R, Vouche M, Sze DY, Hohlastos E, Collins J, Schirmang T, Memon K, Ryu RK, Sato K, Chen R, Gupta R. Cancer concepts and principles: primer for the interventional oncologist—part II. J Vasc Interv Radiol. 2013;24(8):1167–88.
3. Solomon SB, Silverman SG. Imaging in interventional oncology. Radiology. 2010; 257(3):624–40.
4. Arai Y. Clinical trials of interventional oncology. Int J Clin Oncol. 2012;17:301–5.
5. Hoffer FA. Interventional oncology: the future. Pediatr Radiol. 2011;41(Suppl 1):S201–6.
6. Lo CM, Ngan H, Tso WK, et al. Randomized controlled trial of transarterial lipiodol chemoembolization for unresectable hepatocellular carcinoma. Hepatology. 2002;35:1164–71.
7. Kwan SW, Kerlan RK Jr, Sunshine JH. Utilization of interventional oncology treatments in the United States. J Vasc Interv Radiol. 2010;21:1054–60.
8. Liu CY, Chen KF, Chen PJ. Treatment of liver cancer. Cold Spring Harb Perspect Med. 2015;5(9):a021535.
9. Kalva SP, Thabet A, Wicky S. Recent advances in transarterial therapy of primary and secondary liver malignancies. Radiographics. 2008;28(1):101–17.
10. Wang CY, Hu J, Sheth RA, Oklu R. Emerging embolic agents in endovascular embolization: an overview. Progress Biomed Eng. 2020;2(1):012003.
11. Helmberger T. The evolution of interventional oncology in the 21st century. Br J Radiol. 2020;93(1113):20200112.
12. Kanazawa S. Current status of interventional oncology. Int J Clin Oncol. 2012;17(4):299–300.
13. Adam A, Kenny LM. Interventional oncology in multidisciplinary cancer treatment in the 21st century. Nat Rev Clin Oncol. 2015;12(2):105–13.

Chapter 19
Peripheral Vascular Intervention

Eva Liu and Jason Martin

Risk Factors

Modifiable risk factors:

1. Cigarette smoking.
2. Diabetes mellitus.
3. Dyslipidemia.
4. Hypertension.

   Non-modifiable risk factors

1. Advanced age.
2. Male sex, post-menopausal women.
3. Family history/genetics.
4. Socioeconomic status/race.

Cigarette smoking remains one of the strongest risk factors for PAD with the estimated attributable risk to be as high as 76%. Both current and former smokers are at elevated risk for PAD, but smoking cessation can decrease the risk and progression of disease. Active smoking is associated with more severe claudication, increased graft failure, and increased amputation rates (Fig. 19.1).

E. Liu (✉)
Michael G. DeGroote School of Medicine, McMaster University, Hamilton, ON, Canada
e-mail: eva.liu@medportal.ca

J. Martin
Department of Medical Imaging, University of Toronto, Toronto, ON, Canada
e-mail: martin@medportal.ca

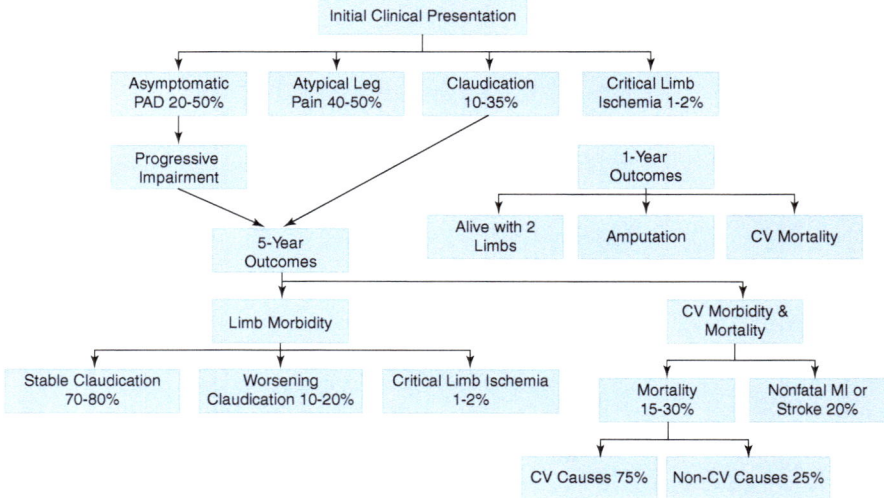

Fig. 19.1 Presentation, evolution, and outcomes in PAD

Differential Diagnosis

The differential diagnosis for leg pain includes arterial claudication, diabetic neuropathy, spinal stenosis, and hip arthritis (Fig. 19.2). Arriving at the correct diagnosis requires careful interviewing and examination of the patient.

Arterial Claudication

Arterial claudication classically presents as a squeezing cramp in the calf or buttock that is precipitated by a predictable distance of walking (e.g., 10–25 steps, 100 m, 200 m) that is relieved with few minutes of rest.

Critical limb ischemia which is a more advanced disease than arterial claudication can present as resting ischemic pain or tissue loss. Resting ischemic pain is characterized by a gnawing pain in the toes that is present at rest. Tissue loss refers to nonhealing ulcers or gangrenous changes in the foot.

Diabetic Neuropathy

Diabetic neuropathy is a difficult diagnosis to distinguish from PAD as some patients can present with bilateral persistent pain in the toes that mimic critical limb ischemia. The sensory deficits as a result of diabetic neuropathy may also make the physical examination results difficult to interpret.

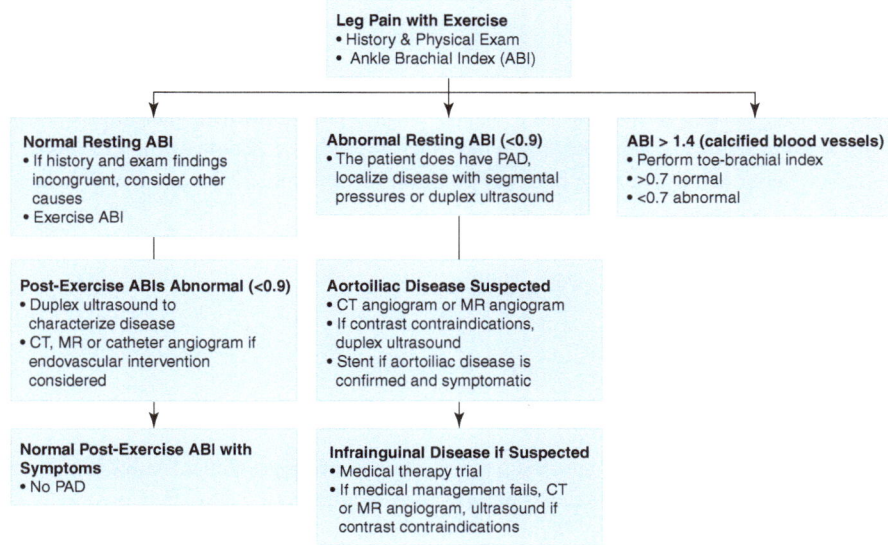

Fig. 19.2 Diagnostic workup of PAD

Noninvasive duplex ultrasound results can be used to correlate the objective findings of stenosis to patient symptoms. Patient symptoms that are out of proportion with the degree of stenosis seen on ultrasound along with history of diabetes are suspicious for diabetic neuropathy. Patient symptoms that are symmetrical in both legs but the stenosis is only seen in one leg along with history of diabetes are also suspicious for diabetic neuropathy.

Nevertheless, both conditions may be present concurrently in the same patient, and it is a diagnostic challenge to determine which factor is the major contributor to the patient's symptoms and whether intervention would be appropriate.

Spinal Stenosis

Spinal stenosis mimics claudication in that both are brought on by exercise and relieved by rest. However, pain caused by spinal stenosis typically radiates down the leg and can be described to be burning in quality which is atypical for arterial claudication. Additionally, spinal stenosis pain is usually positional and can be provoked and alleviated by certain positions of the back. There is also often accompanying back pain that is also affected by the same positions.

Hip Arthritis

Hip arthritis typically presents as pain or ache in the groin region that is exacerbated by walking or weight bearing and relieved with rest. Hip arthritis can improve with physiotherapy or massage therapy which is not typical of claudication. On physical exams, patients may endorse pain with certain movements of the hip which is again atypical of claudication.

Anatomy

General Principles

1. Patients with intermittent claudication should undergo trial of smoking cessation, exercise, and pharmacotherapy. Revascularization can be considered in severe lifestyle-limiting claudication after a patient has failed conservative therapy.
2. Patients with critical limb ischemia presenting with resting ischemic pain and tissue loss should be offered revascularization to restore arterial flow to the foot.
3. Inflow (aortoiliac) and outflow (infrapopliteal) should be assessed before attempted revascularization. Inflow lesions should be revascularized first, followed by outflow lesions if symptoms persist.
4. Patients undergoing revascularization should be aggressively managed for cardiovascular risk factor modification, as myocardial infarction (MI), stroke, and cardiovascular deaths are very high among these individuals.
5. A foot inspection should be performed at every visit, as it is essential to avoid foot amputation.

Indications

Two clear indications exist for revascularization in PAD: critical limb ischemia and claudication that causes functional impairment [1, 2].

Contraindications

No absolute contraindications to using stents in peripheral vessels exist. Renal insufficiency may limit the ability to use iodinated contrast for the procedure. Carbon dioxide angiography could be performed in cases with renal impairment or allergy to contrast medium. Pregnancy contraindicates the use of radiation [1, 2].

Specific Revascularization

General Principles

In endovascular revascularization, the interventionist uses a wire to cross the lesion using either the intraluminal or subintimal approach. The intraluminal approach uses wire and support catheters to find a point of opening through the true lumen. The subintimal approach uses the wire to create a neolumen between the intimal and adventitial layer of the vessel. The interventionist must then penetrate back to the true lumen past the point of the stenosis. After the lesion has been successfully crossed with a wire, percutaneous balloon angioplasty is performed to open the lumen of the vessel. The interventionist must then decide whether or not stents need to be placed based on the degree of residual stenosis, the length of lesion, and the location of lesion. At the end of the procedure, a completion angiogram is performed to visualize the patency of the revascularized vessel.

Iliac Artery Disease [1]

The common iliac artery is an excellent target for endovascular procedures. The stenting initial success rate is >90%, complication rate <2%, and 5-year patency about 80% (Fig. 19.3). Retrospective studies show acceptable rates of primary patency in lesions TASC A-D (Fig. 19.1) (see later for TASC classifications). If claudicating symptoms are thought to be due to iliac disease, noninvasive arterial duplex ultrasound should be the first-line investigation followed by CT angiography with the intent of subsequent percutaneous or open revascularization.

Meta-analysis of six-trials (2116 patients) comparing PTA versus primary stenting showed that no statistically significant differences in procedural complications or 30-day mortality were noted [1]. The stent group showed higher procedural success rates and superior primary patency at 4-year follow-up [1].

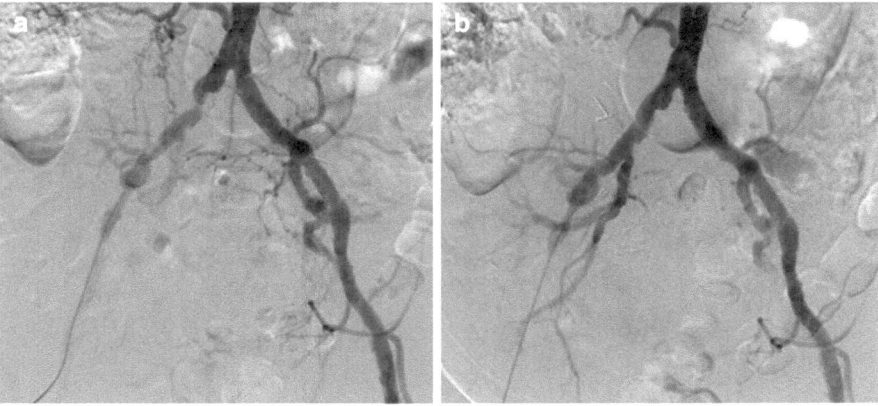

Fig. 19.3 (a) Left common iliac stent and right common iliac artery stenosis. (b) Right common iliac artery stenosis treated by self-expanding stent

Infrainguinal Disease

The benefit of revascularization is less pronounced relative to aortoiliac disease. Excellent results can be achieved with short focal lesions. Longer lesions are associated with lower patency rates over time. Common femoral artery (CFA), superficial femoral artery (SFA), and popliteal artery are all relatively superficial vessels. Sitting, standing, and exertion can affect the patency of these superficial vessels (Fig. 19.4). CFA endarterectomy remains the treatment of choice for CFA lesions due to the

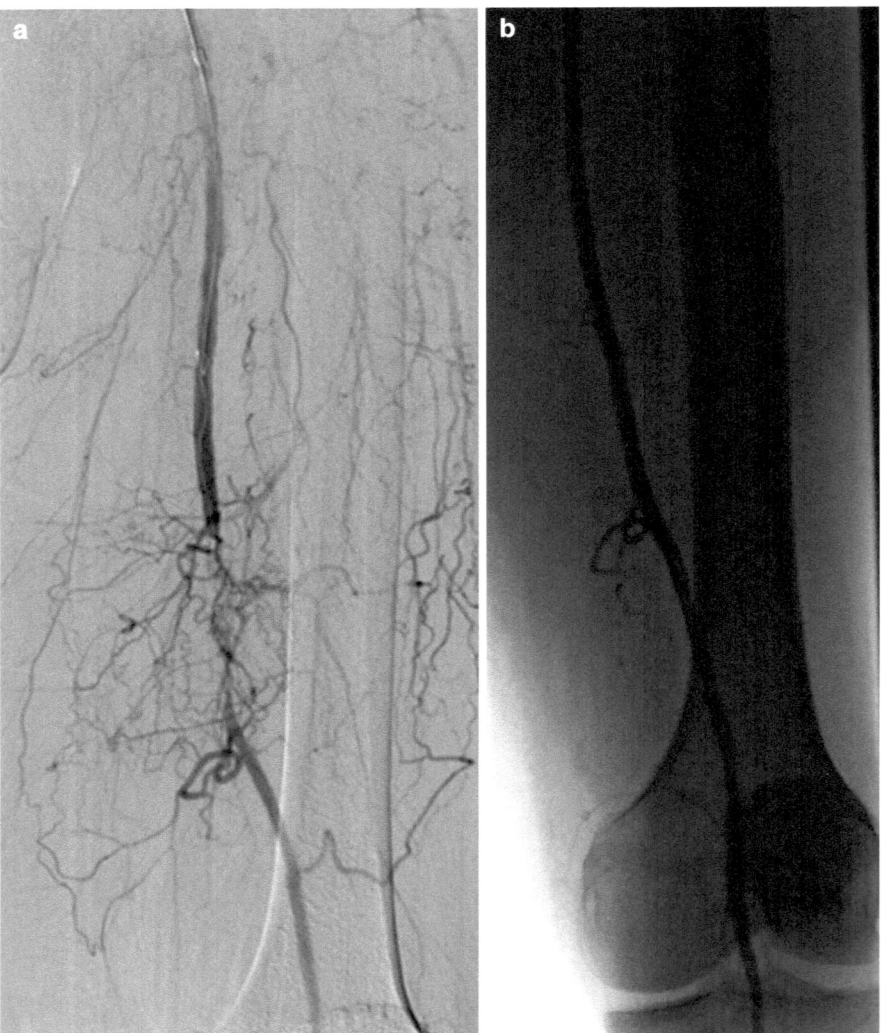

Fig. 19.4 (**a**) Superficial femoral artery occlusion. (**b**) Post-angioplasty and stenting of occluded superficial femoral artery

theoretical risk of stent fracture with hip flexion and the potential loss of a vascular access site [2, 3].

Balloon Angioplasty Versus Stenting of SFA

Balloon angioplasty offers excellent technical success rates, but higher restenosis rates compared to other vascular beds [4–7]. Since balloon-expandable stents are deformed by compression, their use in SFA has been replaced by self-expandable nitinol stents. In short lesions (<5 cm), balloon angioplasty and provisional stenting should be used, and in large lesions (>5 cm), primary stenting is a reasonable choice.

Stent fracture has been linked with early restenosis and occlusion [4]. The highest rate of stent fracture occurs with the use of multiple overlapping long stents, while single short stents have the lowest likelihood of stent fracture [5–7].

Tibial and Peroneal Disease

Unlikely to be the sole cause of functional claudication, tibial and peroneal disease rarely occurs in isolation. Tibial and peroneal disease are common in patients with diabetes and end-stage renal disease. Technical success and patency are reduced, and complications are more common compared to more proximal interventions. Stenting has been shown to have improved patency compared to balloon angioplasty, but reductions in clinical outcomes such as mortality, limb salvage, and other morbidities have not been demonstrated [4–7].

Classification

The classification of vascular disease is based on the Trans-Atlantic Inter Society Consensus (TASC) document on the management of peripheral arterial disease (Figs. 19.5 and 19.6 [8]).

Procedure

Please refer to the chapter on arterial access (Chap. 8) for an overview of the Seldinger technique.

Vascular access is achieved using an 18-gauge needle or micropuncture kit. An angiogram is performed to assess for adequate flow, as well as areas of specific stenosis (Fig. 19.7). A guide wire is used to cross the lesion of concern. The wire

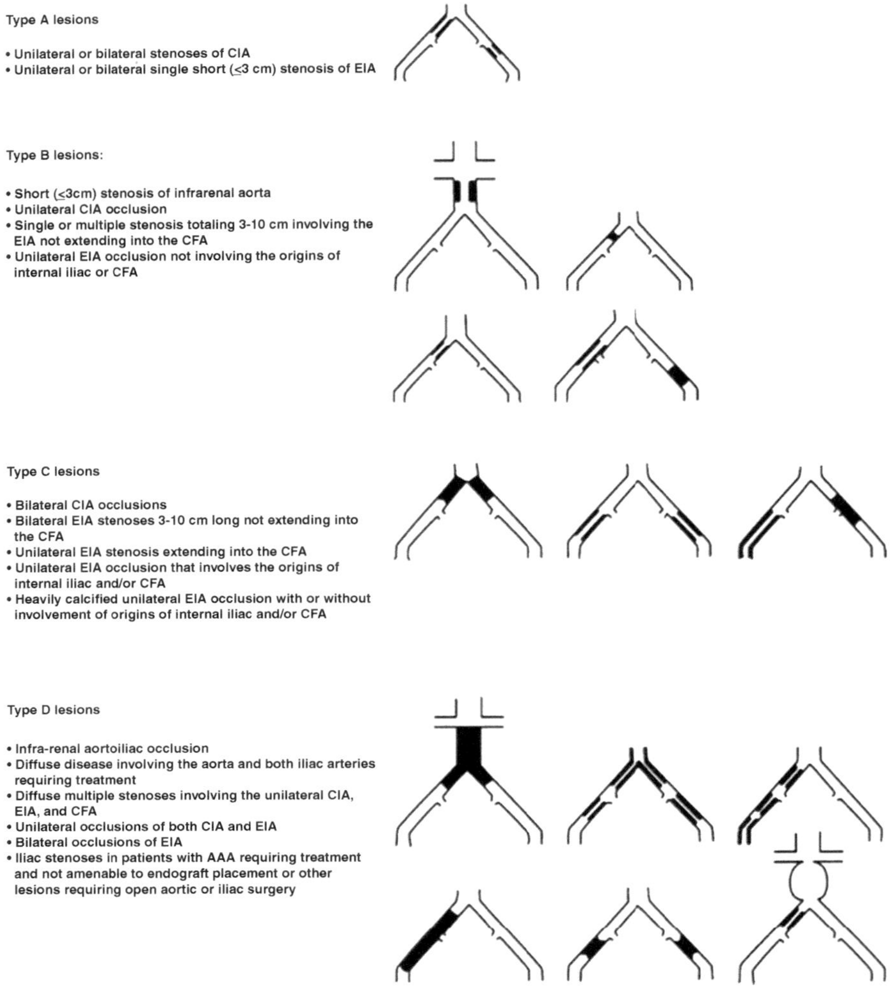

Type A lesions

• Unilateral or bilateral stenoses of CIA
• Unilateral or bilateral single short (≤3 cm) stenosis of EIA

Type B lesions:

• Short (<3cm) stenosis of infrarenal aorta
• Unilateral CIA occlusion
• Single or multiple stenosis totaling 3-10 cm involving the
  EIA not extending into the CFA
• Unilateral EIA occlusion not involving the origins of
  internal iliac or CFA

Type C lesions

• Bilateral CIA occlusions
• Bilateral EIA stenoses 3-10 cm long not extending into
  the CFA
• Unilateral EIA stenosis extending into the CFA
• Unilateral EIA occlusion that involves the origins of
  internal iliac and/or CFA
• Heavily calcified unilateral EIA occlusion with or without
  involvement of origins of internal iliac and/or CFA

Type D lesions

• Infra-renal aortoiliac occlusion
• Diffuse disease involving the aorta and both iliac arteries
  requiring treatment
• Diffuse multiple stenoses involving the unilateral CIA,
  EIA, and CFA
• Unilateral occlusions of both CIA and EIA
• Bilateral occlusions of EIA
• Iliac stenoses in patients with AAA requiring treatment
  and not amenable to endograft placement or other
  lesions requiring open aortic or iliac surgery

Fig. 19.5 TASC II classification of aortoiliac peripheral arterial disease

must be long enough to accommodate the shaft length of the stent device. Choose the right size sheath to allow the insertion of the balloon catheter or stent deployment system as recommended by the manufacturer.

If angioplasty is initially performed, a balloon is placed across the lesion and inflated for 1–2 min, without exceeding the vessel diameter. Residual stenosis >30–40% or flow-limiting intimal dissection prompts the placement of a stent.

Type A Lesions

- Single Stenosis ≤10 cm in Length
- Single Oclusion ≤5 cm in Length

Type B Lesions

- Multiple Lesions (Stenoses or Occlusions),
  Each ≤5 cm
- Single Stenosis or Occlusions ≤15 cm
  Not Involving the Infrageniculate Popliteal Artery
- Single or Multiple Lesions in the Absence
  of continuous Tibial Vessels to Improve Inflow
  for a Distal Bypass
- Heavily Calcified Occlusion ≤5 cm in Length
- Single Popliteal Stenosis

Type C Lesions

- Multiple Stenoses or Occlusions Totaling >15 cm
  With or Without Heavy Calcification
- Recurrent Stenoses or Occlusions That Need
  Treatment After 2 Endovascular Interventions

Type D Lesions

- Chronic Total Occlusions of CFA or SFA
  (>20 cm, Involving the Popliteal Artery)
- Chronic Total Occlusion of Popliteal Artery
  and Proximal Trifurcation Vessels

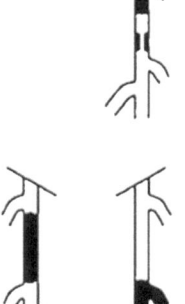

Fig. 19.6 TASC II classification of femoropopliteal peripheral arterial disease

Balloon-expandable stents must match the vessel diameter, but self-expandable stents may be upsized to maintain radial force on the vessel wall. Predilection with a smaller balloon can help pass the stent device, as balloon-expandable stents are more rigid and less trackable than self-expanding stents.

The length of the stent should cover the length of the lesion. If multiple stents are required, 1–2 cm of overlap should be used and stents placed distally first then extending proximally.

Angiography is performed to assess the result of the intervention, and distal imaging is useful to rule out embolization following the intervention.

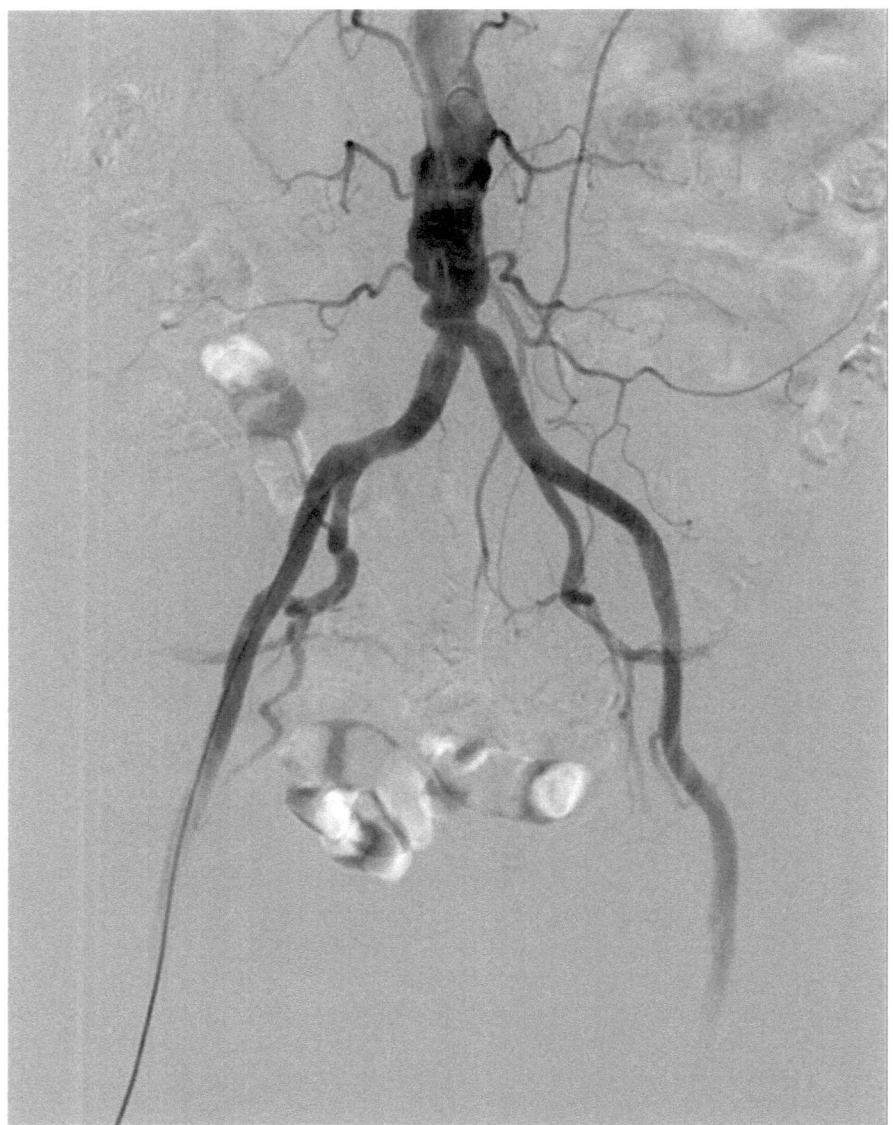

Fig. 19.7 Aortogram with catheter in distal abdominal aorta

Complications

Complications include:

- Bleeding (hematoma or pseudoaneurysm) at the puncture site.
- Infection.
- Dissection of vessel.

- Contrast nephropathy.
- Distal embolization.
- Stent fracture.
- In-stent thrombosis or restenosis.
- Arterial rupture.
- Arterial spasm.

Outcomes

Femoropopliteal Stenting Versus PTA

Variables associated with favorable femoropopliteal PTA include claudication, non-diabetic patients, proximal short lesions, good distal runoff, lack of residual stenosis on post-PTA angiogram, and ABI improvement by >0.1 [9–11].

Primary patency rates for femoropopliteal PTA are 47–86% at 1 year, 42–60% at 3 years, and 41–58% at 5 years [9–16]. For femoropopliteal stenting, patency rates are 22–86% at 1 year and 18–72% at 3 years [17–19].

The literature surrounding drug-eluting stents in the femoropopliteal artery is still developing. The 18-month results from the SIROCCO trial showed no restenosis in the slow-release sirolimus-eluting stent group, compared to the rates of 33 and 30 % in the rapid drug-eluting stent group and uncoated stent group, respectively [20].

Iliac Artery PTA Versus Stenting

For iliac artery PTA, the technical and initial clinical success is >90%, and 5-year patency rates range between 54 and 92% [12, 21–26]. Stenting of iliac arteries provides a 3-year patency rate of 41–92% for stenoses and 64–85% for occlusions [27–44]. Stents do appear to improve the results of iliac PTA without an increased complication rate. Factors associated with decreased patency rates include poor quality of runoff vessels, severity of ischemia, and extended length of diseased segments [12, 21–44].

Infrapopliteal Stenting Versus PTA

PTA is mainly used in the setting of critical limb ischemia. Clinical success is more important than angiographic improvement as collateral flow may be enough to preserve tissue perfusion if there is no subsequent injury (Fig. 19.8 [45]). The primary

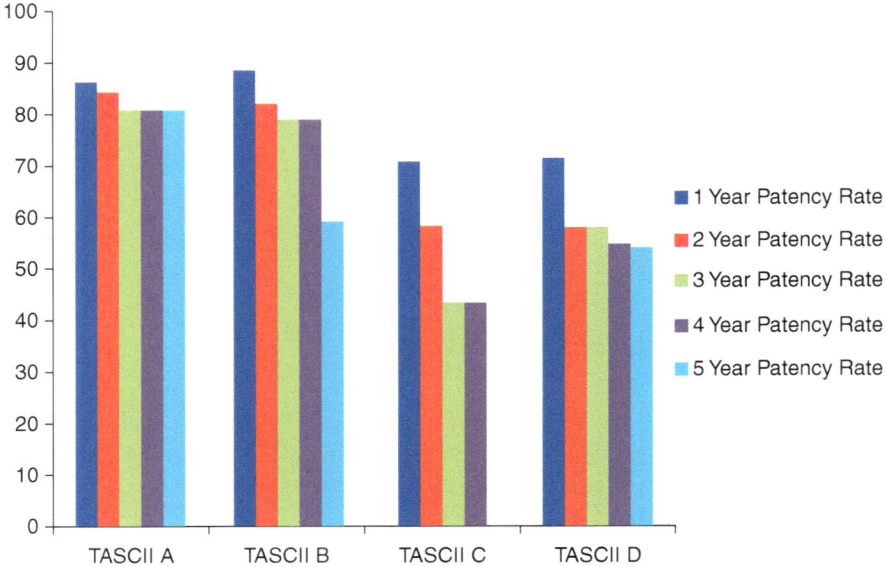

Fig. 19.8 Femoropopliteal intervention. Primary potency among TASC II classifications. Retrospective study involving 639 limbs in 511 patients using self-expanding nitinol stents [45]

patency rate for PTA in infrapopliteal vessels ranges from 40 to 81% at 1 year and 78% at 2 years [46–49]. Limb salvage rate is higher at 77–89% at 1 year [46–49]. The presence of diabetes and renal failure are risk factors for limb loss in this setting [46, 50].

Intimal Hyperplasia

Vascular injury after intraluminal manipulation results in the thickening of the tunica intima of a blood vessel—intimal hyperplasia (IH). This contributes to a high rate of restenosis in diffuse segmental stenosis or when multiple stents are placed [17, 51]. Animal studies reveal that slow flow promotes thrombus deposition as well as more pronounced IH [52, 53]. The rate of IH is related to the caliber of arteries as well. Surface thrombus reduces the effective circulation in smaller arteries more markedly, leading to increased restenosis rates in smaller caliber arteries. When this hypothesis was studied, stent restenosis rates were found to increase with decreased vessel caliber: 4% in the proximal SFA, 10% in the mid-segment of the SFA, and >18% in the distal SFA [51]. Metal stents used were made smaller to minimize restenosis through improvements in mesh design [54].

Several interventions or modifications are currently being explored to improve rates of IH. Modifications of the polymer cover of stent grafts may improve patency. Graft pore size modifications and Dacron or PTFE-covered stent grafts are also being explored [55–57]. Stents with drug carrier systems to inhibit IH are also being investigated. The SIROCCO study examines a self-expanding nitinol stent coated with a polymer containing sirolimus (a lactone with immunosuppressive activity) [58].

General Principles: Procedure Preparation

Note: these principles are meant for local and not general anesthesia

- Required the day before the procedure: focused history and physical examination, focused labs (CBC/electrolytes, coagulation profile with PT/PTT).
- Vitals pre-, intra- and post procedures, particularly for individuals taking cardiac medication.
- Fasting/NPO status for an appropriate duration before the procedure.
- Confirmation of appropriate adherence to anticoagulation discontinuation instructions as per internal medicine/hematology recommendations.

Acknowledgment We would like to thank Dr. Jason Martin for his contributions to this chapter (information given on first page of chapter).

References

1. Bosch JL, Hunink MG. Meta-analysis of the results of percutaneous transluminal angioplasty and stent placement for aortoiliac occlusive disease. Radiology. 1997;204:87–96.
2. Mukherjee D, Inahara T. Endarterectomy as the procedure of choice for atherosclerotic occlusive lesions of the common femoral artery. Am J Surg. 1989;157:498–500.
3. Springhorn ME, Kinney M, Littooy FN, et al. Inflow atherosclerotic disease localized to the common femoral artery: treatment and outcome. Ann Vasc Surg. 1991;5:234–40.
4. Scheinert D, Scheinert S, Piorkowski C, Braunlich S, Ulrich M, Biamino G, et al. Prevalence and impact of stent fractures after femoropopliteal stenting. J Am Coll Cardiol. 2005;45:312–5.
5. Krankenberg H, Schluter M, Steinkamp HJ, Burgelin K, Scheinert D, Schulte KL, et al. Nitinol stent implantation versus percutaneous transluminal angioplasty in superficial femoral artery lesions up to 10 cm in length: the femoral artery stenting trial (FAST). Circulation. 2007;116:285–92.
6. Laird JR, Katzen BT, Scheinert D, Lammer J, Carpenter J, Buchbinder M, et al. Nitinol stent implantation versus balloon angioplasty for lesions in the superficial femoral artery and proximal popliteal artery: twelve-month results from the RESILIENT randomized trial. Circ Cardiovasc Interv. 2010;3:267–76.
7. Duda SH, Bosiers M, Lammer J, Scheinert D, Zeller T, Oliva V, et al. Drug-eluting and bare nitinol stents for the treatment of atherosclerotic lesions in the superficial femoral artery: long-term results from the SIROCCO trial. J Endovasc Ther. 2006;13:701–10.
8. Norgren L, Hiatt WR, Dormandy JA, Nehler MR, Harris KA, Fowkes FG, et al. Inter-society consensus for the management of peripheral arterial disease (TASC II). Eur J Vasc Endovasc Surg. 2007;33:S1–75.
9. Capek P, McLean GK, Berkowitz HD. Femoropopliteal angioplasty: factors influencing long-term success. Circulation. 1991;83(suppl 2):I70–80.

10. Johnston KW. Femoral and popliteal arteries: reanalysis of results of balloon angioplasty. Radiology. 1992;183:767–71.
11. Matsi PJ, Manninen HI, Vanninen RL, et al. Femoropopliteal angioplasty in patients with claudication: primary and secondary patency in 140 limbs with 1–3 years follow up. Radiology. 1994;191:727–33.
12. Jeans WD, Amstrong S, Cole SEA, et al. Fate of patients undergoing transluminal angioplasty for lower-limb ischemia. Radiology. 1990;177:559–64.
13. Murray JG, Apthorp LA, Wilkins RA. Long-segment (>10 cm) femoropopliteal angioplasty: improved technical success and long-term patency. Radiology. 1995;195:158–62.
14. Gallino A, Mahler F, Probst P, et al. Percutaneous transluminal angioplasty of the arteries of the lower limbs: a 5-year follow-up. Circulation. 1984;70(4):619–23.
15. Krepel VM, van Andel GJ, van Erp WF, et al. Percutaneous transluminal angioplasty of the femoropopliteal artery: initial and long-term results. Radiology. 1985;156(2):325–8.
16. Hunink MG, Donaldson MC, Meyerovitz MF, et al. Risks and benefits of femoropopliteal percutaneous balloon angioplasty. J Vasc Surg. 1993;17(1):183–92.
17. Gray BH, Olin JW. Limitations of percutaneous transluminal angioplasty with stenting for femoropopliteal arterial occlusive disease. Semin Vasc Surg. 1997;10:8–16.
18. Strecker EPS, Boos IBL, Gottmann D. Femoropopliteal artery stent-placement: evaluation of long-term success. Radiology. 1997;205:375–83.
19. Rosenfield K, Schainfeld R, Pieczek A, et al. Restenosis of endovascular stents from stent compression. J Am Coll Cardiol. 1997;29:328–38.
20. Duda SH, Wiesinger B, Richter GM, et al. Sirolimus-eluting stents in SFA obstructions: long-term SIROCCO trial results. CIRSE 2003 annual meeting and postgraduate course. Main Programme and Abstracts: abstr 35.3.2, p. 157.
21. van Andel GJ, van Erp WF, Krepel VM, et al. Percutaneous transluminal dilatation of the iliac artery: long-term results. Radiology. 1985;156:321–4.
22. Blankensteijn JD, van Broonhoven TJ, Lampmann L. Role of percutaneous transluminal angioplasty in aorto-iliac reconstruction. J Cardiovasc Surg (Torino). 1986;27:466–8.
23. Tegtmeyer CJ, Hartwell GD, Selby JB, et al. Results and complications of angioplasty in aortoiliac disease. Circulation. 1991;83(Suppl 2):53–60.
24. Jorgensen B, Skovgaard N, Norgard J, et al. Percutaneous transluminal angioplasty in 226 iliac artery stenoses: role of the superficial femoral artery for clinical success. Vasa. 1992;21:382–6.
25. Johnston KW. Iliac arteries: reanalysis of results of balloon angioplasty. Radiology. 1993;186:207–12.
26. Rholl KS. Percutaneous aortoiliac intervention in vascular disease. In: Baum S, Pentecost MJ, editors. Abram's angiography, interventional radiology, vol. III. Boston: Little, Brown; 1997. p. 225–61.
27. Palmaz JC, Laborde JC, Rivera FJ, et al. Stenting of iliac arteries with the Palmaz stent: experience from a multicentric trial. Cardiovasc Intervent Radiol. 1992;15:291–7.
28. Vorwerk D, Gunther RW. Stent placement in iliac arterial lesions: three years of clinical experience with the Wallstent. Cardiovasc Intervent Radiol. 1992;15:285–90.
29. Strecker EP, Hagen P, Liermann D, et al. Iliac and femoropopliteal vascular occlusive disease treated with flexible tantalum stents. Cardiovasc Intervent Radiol. 1993;16:158–64.
30. Wolf YG, Schatz RA, Knowles HJ, et al. Initial experience with the Palmaz stent for aortoiliac stenoses. Ann Vasc Surg. 1993;7:254–61.
31. Martin EC, Katzen BT, Benenati JF, et al. Multicenter trial of the Wallstent in iliac and femoral arteries. J Vasc Interv Radiol. 1995;6:843–9.
32. Vorwerk D, Guenther R, Schurmann K, et al. Aortic and iliac stenoses: follow-up results of stent placement after insufficient balloon angioplasty in 118 cases. Radiology. 1996;198:45–8.
33. Murphy TP, Webb MS, Lambiase RE, et al. Percutaneous revascularization of complex iliac artery stenoses and occlusions with use of Wallstent: three-year experience. J Vasc Interv Radiol. 1996;7:21–7.
34. Tetteroo E, van der Graaf Y, Bosch JL, The Dutch Iliac Stent Trial Study Group, et al. Randomised comparison of primary stent placement versus primary angioplasty followed by selective stent placement in patients with iliac artery occlusive disease. Lancet. 1998;351:1153–9.

35. Treiman GS, Schneider PA, Lawrence PF, et al. Does stent placement improve the results of ineffective or complicated iliac artery angioplasty? J Vasc Surg. 1998;28:104–12.
36. Hassen-Khodja R, Sala F, Declemy S, et al. Value of stent placement during percutaneous transluminal angioplasty of the iliac arteries. J Cardiovasc Surg (Torino). 2001;42:369–74.
37. Vorwerk D, Guenther R, Schurmann K, et al. Primary stent placement for chronic iliac artery occlusions: follow-up results in 103 patients. Radiology. 1995;194:745–9.
38. Dyett JF, Gaines PA, Nicholson AA, Cleveland T, et al. Treatment of chronic iliac artery occlusions by means of endovascular stent placement. J Vasc Interv Radiol. 1997;8:349–53.
39. Henry M, Amor M, Ethevenot G, et al. Percutaneous treatment of iliac occlusions: long-term follow-up in 105 patients. J Endovasc Surg. 1998;5:228–35.
40. Ballard JL, Bergan JJ, Singh P, et al. Aortoiliac stent deployment versus surgical reconstruction: analysis of outcome and cost. J Vasc Surg. 1998;28:94–101.
41. Scheinert D, Schroder M, Ludwig J, et al. Stent-supported recanalization of chronic iliac occlusions. Am J Med. 2001;110:708–15.
42. Uher P, Nyman U, Lindh M, et al. Long-term results for stenting chronic iliac occlusions. J Endovasc Ther. 2002;9:67–75.
43. Funovics MA, Lackner B, Cejna M, et al. Predictors of long-term results after treatment of iliac artery obliteration by transluminal angioplasty and stent placement. Cardiovasc Intervent Radiol. 2002;25:397–402.
44. Carnevale FC, De Blas M, Merino S, et al. Percutaneous endovascular treatment of chronic iliac artery occlusion. Cardiovasc Intervent Radiol. 2004;27:447–52.
45. Soga Y, Lida O, Hirano K, Yokoi H, Nanto S, Nobuyoshi M. Mid-term clinical outcome and predictors of vessel patency after femoropopliteal stenting with self-expandable nitinol stent. J Vasc Surg. 2010;52:608–15.
46. Soder HK, Manninen HI, Jaakkola P, et al. Prospective trial of infrapopliteal artery balloon angioplasty for critical limb ischemia. J Vasc Interv Radiol. 2000;11:1021–31.
47. Lofberg AM, Karacagil S, Ljungman C, et al. Percutaneous transluminal angioplasty of the femoropopliteal arteries in limbs with chronic critical limb ischemia. J Vasc Surg. 2001;34:114–21.
48. Boyer L, Therre T, Garcier JM, et al. Infra-popliteal percutaneous transluminal angioplasty limb salvage. Acta Radiol. 2000;41:73–7.
49. London NJ, Varty K, Sayers RD, et al. Percutaneous transluminal angioplasty for lower-limb critical ischemia. Br J Surg. 1996;83:135–6.
50. Vainio E, Salenius JP, Lepantalo M, et al. Endovascular surgery for chronic lower limb ischemia. Factors predicting immediate outcome on the basis of a nationwide vascular registry. Ann Chir Gynaecol. 2001;90:86–91.
51. Henry M, Amor M, Ethevenot G, et al. Palmaz stent placement in iliac and femoropopliteal arteries: primary and secondary patency in 310 patients with 2–4-year follow-up. Radiology. 1995;197:167–74.
52. Kauffmann GW, et al. Four years' experience with a balloon-expandable endoprosthesis: experimental and clinical application. Radiologe. 1991;31:202–9.
53. Richter GM, Palmaz JC, Noeldge G, et al. Relationship between blood flow, thrombus, and neointima in stents. J Vasc Interv Radiol. 1999;10:598–604.
54. Palmaz JC. Balloon expandable intravascular stent. Am J Roentgenol. 1988;150:1263–9.
55. Golden MA, Hanson SR, Kirkman TR, et al. Healing of polytetrafluoroethylene arterial grafts is influenced by graft porosity. J Vasc Surg. 1990;11:838–45.
56. Ahmadi R, Schillinger M, Maca T, et al. Femoropopliteal arteries: immediate and long-term results with a Dacron-covered stent-graft. Radiology. 2002;223:345–50.
57. Jahnke T, Andersen R, Muller-Hulsbeck S, et al. Hemobahn stent-grafts for treatment of femoropoliteal arterial obstructions: midterm results of a prospective trial. J Vasc Interv Radiol. 2003;14:41–55.
58. Duda SH, Pusich B, Richter G, et al. Sirolimus-eluting stents for the treatment of obstructive superficial femoral artery disease. Circulation. 2002;106:1505–9.

Chapter 20
Lymphatic Interventions

Anna Hwang

Diagnostic Lymphangiography

Before any therapeutic interventions are attempted, the lymphatic leak must be localized. Diagnostic methods include pedal lymphangiography, intranodal lymphangiography, magnetic resonance (MR) lymphangiography, and direct contrast-enhanced MR lymphangiography (DCRML).

Pedal Lymphangiography

Pedal lymphangiography is the oldest form of lymphatic imaging and involves injection of Lipiodol, a lipid-based contrast agent, into the lymphatic vessels within the dorsum of the foot.

- This procedure requires a high level of technical skill, as the dorsum of the foot must be incised and its lymphatic vessels carefully exposed and cannulated [1].
- Lipiodol is injected into the cannulated vessels and monitored with intermittent fluoroscopy as it travels up the legs and into the central lymphatics [1].
- The site of any leaks are determined by observing extravasation of the contrast agent fluoroscopically.
- Pedal lymphangiography is time-consuming, as the contrast agent can take several hours to reach the area of interest [2].
- Complications include pedal incision site injury, infection, leg edema, and mild pulmonary embolism [1, 3].

A. Hwang (✉)
Michael G. DeGroote School of Medicine, McMaster University, Hamilton, ON, Canada
e-mail: anna.hwang@medportal.ca

© The Author(s), under exclusive license to Springer Nature   221
Switzerland AG 2022
S. Athreya, M. Albahhar (eds.), *Demystifying Interventional Radiology*,
https://doi.org/10.1007/978-3-031-12023-7_20

Intranodal Lymphangiography

Since 2012, intranodal lymphangiography has largely replaced pedal lymphangiography because of its higher success rates and relative ease of use [4, 5].

- First, a suitable inguinal lymph node is located by ultrasound and punctured with a 26-gauge needle.
- Once proper positioning of the needle is confirmed, a total of 3–6 mL of Lipiodol is injected into the lymph node and monitored with fluoroscopy [6].
- Because the inguinal lymph nodes are closer to the abdomen and thorax than the lymphatic vessels of the foot, the contrast reaches its target location more rapidly and is less diluted by the time it reaches the site.
- On average, it takes approximately 40 min to visualize the thoracic duct after injection of Lipiodol [7].
- Complications include pain, infection, and mild pulmonary embolism [1, 8].

Non-Contrast MR Lymphangiography

Non-contrast T2-weighted MR lymphangiography is a noninvasive method useful for imaging the central and peripheral lymphatics. Non-bloody, slow-moving fluids produce a high T2 signal, allowing for visualization of different parts of the peripheral lymphatic system, as well as segments of the central lymphatics [5]. However, this method does not provide any useful information about lymphatic flow. Additionally, without a contrast agent, smaller lymphatic ducts are hard to discern [5].

Dynamic Contrast-Enhanced MR Lymphangiography

DCMRL is a relatively new technique, in which a gadolinium-based contrast agent is injected into inguinal lymph nodes and imaged with MR. Previously, contrast agents were injected intradermally or subcutaneously, which was useful for imaging the extremities but ineffective for imaging the central lymphatics due to dilution of the contrast agent:

- DCMRL bypasses the lower extremities, resulting in fast and effective imaging of the central lymphatic ducts [5].
- The gadolinium-based contrast agent used in DCMRL is less viscous than Lipiodol, allowing for more sensitive detection of abdominal leaks [1].
- DCMRL can be used as an alternative to lymphangiography and is safe for all patients who have no contraindications to MR (e.g., implanted electronic devices).
- Complications are typically minor and include infection, localized pain, and contrast reaction [5].

Therapeutic Procedures

In about 50% of cases, invasive lymphangiography itself is therapeutic, and no further treatment is needed [2]. However, in refractory cases, sclerotherapy or embolization techniques are required to control lymphatic leaks.

Sclerotherapy

Sclerotherapy uses sclerosing agents such as ethanol, acetic acid, povidone–iodine, doxycycline, or bleomycin to obstruct the site of leakage:

- Commonly used adjunctively to treat localized cystic lesions of lymphatic fluid [9].
- Sclerosants are injected into the cysts percutaneously, then drained after a few hours.
- Sclerosants act by causing inflammation and damage to adjacent tissues, with the resultant inflammatory response helping to collapse and fill the cavity.
- Complications include skin blistering, ulceration, swelling, scarring, pain, and nerve injury [10].

Embolization

Embolization techniques typically involve injection of the target site with coils and glue [such as *n*-Butyl-2-cyanoacrylate (NBCA)], after the site has been located by lymphangiography. The coils provide a framework on which the glue polymerizes, resulting in mechanical blockage of the leak [11]. There are several different techniques for embolization.

Lymphopseudoaneurysm Embolization

A lymphopseudoaneurysm is a small, contained collection of extravasated lymphatic fluid [4]:

- Lymphopseudoaneurysms can be punctured with a 21-gauge needle connected to a small syringe.
- After a test injection of Lipiodol confirms that the correct site was punctured, a glue mixture of NCBA and Lipiodol is injected to completely fill the lymphopseudoaneurysm.
- The entire procedure is guided by fluoroscopy or computerized tomography (CT) [4].

Closest Upstream Lymph Node Embolization

With this technique, the lymph node closest to the site of the leak is used as the injection point for an embolizing agent.

- The target lymph node is located by lymphangiography and can be directly punctured with a 22- to 25-gauge needle under fluoroscopy or CT guidance [1].
- After the puncture, test Lipiodol can be injected to gauge the distance between the lymph node and the point of extravasation. If the interventional radiologist decides that the lymph node is too far from the leakage, such that the embolizing agent would prematurely polymerize, a different lymph node would be selected.
- After an appropriate lymph node is located, a glue mixture of Lipiodol and NBCA is injected and fills the draining lymphatics [4].

Direct Upstream Lymphatic Vessel Embolization

The lymphatic vessel from which the leak originates can also be a target for embolization.

- Following localization by lymphangiography, the vessel is punctured under fluoroscopic guidance with a 21-gauge needle [4].
- Using the Seldinger technique, a short guidewire is inserted through the access needle, and the sheath of a dilator is passed over the guidewire to maintain access to the lymphatic vessel.
- Test Lipiodol can be injected to ensure the vessel was cannulated appropriately. Then, a glue mixture of NBCA and Lipiodol is injected into the vessel [4].

Complications of embolization may include transient pain, pulmonary embolism (usually mild), leg swelling, abdominal swelling, and diarrhea [1, 9].

Chylothorax

Chylothorax occurs when chylous fluid leaks into the pleural space and is commonly due to thoracic duct injury following surgery. Other causes of chylothorax include lymphoma, lung cancer, and tuberculosis. The thoracic duct is the largest lymph vessel in the body and carries lymph fluid from the hepatic and enteral lymphatic networks, as well as from the lower extremities [2]. The lymph flowing through the thoracic duct is chylous, meaning that it contains high concentrations of proteins and fat carried over from the enteral and hepatic lymphatic networks. A chylothorax can be life-threatening due to loss of essential proteins, fats, electrolytes, and nutrients [2].

Thoracic duct embolization is a well-established treatment for chylothorax

- After visualization of the thoracic duct and identification of the site of leakage, a microwire is inserted into the duct under fluoroscopy [4].
- Lipiodol is injected into the duct to confirm the point of extravasation.
- Finally, coils and glue are injected to provide mechanical occlusion of the leak [7].

Chylous Ascites

Chylous ascites is an uncommon complication usually caused by trauma to lymphatic vessels from abdominal or pelvic surgery. Other causes include malignancy, cirrhosis, infection, and inflammatory conditions affecting the lymphatic system [1].

When the ascites is refractory to conservative management, interventional radiology becomes involved.

- First, the site of the leak is determined. In some cases, the location of the leak is difficult to visualize by intranodal lymphangiography, and use of dynamic contrast-enhanced MR lymphangiography is required [1].
- When lymphangiography is not by itself therapeutic, lymphatic embolization is employed.
- Embolizing agents can be injected into the closest lymph node to the leak or directly injected into the leaking vessel itself. If injecting the embolizing agent into the nearest lymph node, a mixture of Lipiodol and NBCA glue is used. If targeting the leaking vessel directly, coils and NBCA glue are used [1].

Lymphocele

A lymphocele is a collection of lymphatic fluid surrounded by a fibrotic wall, often arising as a complication of lymphadenectomy from pelvic or retroperitoneal surgery [2]. Lymphoceles are often asymptomatic, but in some cases may cause infection or compression of other structures.

Lymphoceles can be easily drained by a percutaneous catheter, but commonly re-expand after drainage [2].

- Sclerosants may be injected into the lymphocele cavity after percutaneous drainage. Ethanol and povidone–iodine are commonly used sclerosants [9].
- If the lymphocele is refractory to this treatment, embolization techniques are used. Large lymphoceles in particular are more susceptible to dilution of the sclerosing agent and may require embolization of the feeding vessel(s) [9].
- Drainage is then monitored in the days following the procedure [9].

References

1. Nadolski GJ, Chauhan NR, Itkin M. Lymphangiography and lymphatic embolization for the treatment of refractory chylous ascites. Cardiovasc Intervent Radiol. 2018;41:415–23. https://doi.org/10.1007/s00270-017-1856-1.
2. Majdalany BS, El-Haddad G. Contemporary lymphatic interventions for post-operative lymphatic leaks. Transl Androl Urol. 2020;9(Suppl 1):S104–13. https://doi.org/10.21037/tau.2019.08.15.
3. Kim PH, Tsauo J, Shin JH. Lymphatic interventions for chylothorax: a systematic review and meta-analysis. J Vasc Interv Radiol. 2018;29:194–202. https://doi.org/10.1016/j.jvir.2017.10.006.
4. Hur S, Shin JH, Lee IJ, et al. Early experience in the management of postoperative lymphatic leakage using lipiodol lymphangiography and adjunctive glue embolization. J Vasc Interv Radiol. 2016;27:1177–86. https://doi.org/10.1016/j.jvir.2016.05.011.
5. Dori Y. Novel lymphatic imaging techniques. Tech Vasc Interv Radiol. 2016;4:255–61. https://doi.org/10.1053/j.tvir.2016.10.002.
6. Nadolski GJ, Itkin M. Feasibility of ultrasound-guided intranodal lymphangiogram for thoracic duct embolization. J Vasc Interv Radiol. 2012;23:613–6. https://doi.org/10.1016/j.jvir.2012.01.078.
7. Inoue M, Nakatsuka S, Yashiro H, et al. Lymphatic intervention for various types of lymphorrhea: access and treatment. Radiographics. 2016;36:2199–211. https://doi.org/10.1148/rg.2016160053.
8. Syed LH, Georgiades CS, Hart VL. Lymphangiography: a case study. Semin Intervent Radiol. 2007;24:106–10. https://doi.org/10.1055/s-2007-971180.
9. Baek Y, Won JH, Chang SJ, et al. Lymphatic embolization for the treatment of pelvic lymphoceles: preliminary experience in five patients. J Vasc Interv Radiol. 2016;27:1170–6. https://doi.org/10.1016/j.jvir.2016.04.011.
10. Alomari AI, Karian VE, Lord DJ, et al. Percutaneous sclerotherapy for lymphatic malformations: a retrospective analysis of patient-evaluated improvement. J Vasc Interv Radiol. 2006;17(10):1639–48. https://doi.org/10.1097/01.RVI.0000239104.78390.E5.
11. Itkin M. Interventional treatment of pulmonary anomalies. Tech Vasc Interv Radiol. 2016;19(4):299–304. https://doi.org/10.1053/j.tvir.2016.10.005.

Chapter 21
Structured Reporting in IR

Ruqqiyah Rana and Ibrahim Mohammad Nadeem

Headings and Categories

Structured reporting, as elucidated above, simply refers to a standardized way of documenting medical information; there are indeed a diverse range of reporting methods which may be described as "structured." In essence, such reports should include the following headings: type of examination, clinical history, indication, comparison, technique, findings, and impression [1]. While most non-structured IR reports include each of these elements, they often do so in a narrative prose style, with variability in length, headings, flow, and level of detail; as a result, valuable data is often lost due to the lack of uniformity [2].

More advanced structured reports may include subsections within the "findings" category; specific organs may be categorically described and the relevant anatomy systematically and thoroughly reviewed [1]. Reports such as these, with multi-layered data entry, may be best compiled with the aid of report templates, such as those available from the SIR [3].

Data Entry

Structured reporting templates are specific to the procedure being reported and contain within them a variety of methods to enter data. Common methods can include picking from drop-down lists and entering free text under pre-written headings, both of which can be updated manually by the user to increase specificity [4].

R. Rana (✉) · I. M. Nadeem
Michael G. DeGroote School of Medicine, McMaster University, Hamilton, ON, Canada
e-mail: ruqqiyah.rana@medportal.ca; ibrahim.nadeem@medportal.ca

Structured templates available through SIR can be used with any voice recognition software and can be created with xml or rich text format [4]. 31 procedure-specific reports are currently available, updated annually to reflect current guidelines [4].

Advantages

Structured reports remain the cornerstone for efficient reporting and enable both improved patient outcomes and increased ease of access to clinical data required for quality improvement and performance measures [2]. Importantly, the widespread use of structured reports in and among radiologists and referring clinicians improves communicability and reduces diagnostic error [1]. Further, there is an increase in translatability and consistency across specific procedural reports, as templates can be created and accessed for disease-specific interventions [1]. The inclusion of specific standardized headings and the requirement of reporting under each heading allows for comprehensiveness and completion in medical records, as well as ease of access for referring physicians [1]. Finally, the consistent use of systematic reporting increases the efficiency of quality improvement studies and data extraction for research purposes [1, 4].

Disadvantages

Despite the benefits and well-documented advantages of structured reporting in both clinical and research settings, implementation on an international level remains a challenge. Given the initial increase in time requirement and resource intensity, this method of reporting is not popular with all radiologists [1, 2]. The initial learning curve required for populating templates, rather than narrating prose-style, also detracts from the appeal of structured reports; there may be a perceived initial decrease in productivity and efficiency [2]. Further, the adoption of a template with pre-set headings may decrease the flow associated with a natural reporting style and decrease comprehension and understanding of various report elements [2].

References

1. Ganeshan D, Duong PA, Probyn L, Lenchik L, McArthur TA, Retrouvey M, Ghobadi EH, Desouches SL, Pastel D, Francis IR. Structured reporting in radiology. Acad Radiol. 2018;25(1):66–73.
2. Durack JC. The value proposition of structured reporting in interventional radiology. Am J Roentgenol. 2014;203(4):734–8. https://doi.org/10.2214/AJR.14.13112.

3. Society of Interventional Radiology (SIR) and SIR Foundation. Standardized report—dialysis fistula interventions (version 3). 2019. https://sir.personifycloud.com/PersonifyEBusiness/Default.aspx?tabid=251&productId=107725790. Accessed 7 Oct 2021.
4. Society of Interventional Radiology. Frequently asked questions about standardized reports. 2022. https://www.sirweb.org/globalassets/aasociety-of-interventional-radiology-home-page/practice-resources/macra-pdf/frequently-asked-questions-about-standardized-reports%2D%2D031317.pdf. Accessed 7 Oct 2021.
5. Society of Interventional Radiology. VIRTEX SIR Data Registry. 2022. https://www.sirweb.org/virtex. Accessed 10 Oct 2021.

Chapter 22
Role of Technology in IR

Ruqqiyah Rana and Eva Liu

The Future of Technology in IR [1]

Provided in Chapters 1–6 on common instruments and tools in IR is a brief glimpse into the current practice in this rapidly evolving field. The current practice of imaging technology is beyond the scope of this chapter and can be more thoroughly understood by reviewing Chapters 1–6. The more recent advances are being brought about by sophisticated changes in the imaging technology used, automation of procedures and the use of robotics, procedural techniques (building on the established techniques and principles outlined above), and even artificial intelligence [1].

Imaging

The advances seen in the field of imaging focus on the mitigation of radiation exposure harm and enhancing visualization of 3D anatomical structures through a 2D imaging modality [1, 2]. Fiber optic real shape (FORS), tested at the University Medical Center in Utrecht, Netherlands, alleviates the need for repeated catheterization and radiographic exposure for standard imaging [2]. Instead, a single catheter with light-sensing technology is used to replace X-ray imaging and can depict anatomical structures on a large screen in a 3D format. Although the technology at this stage only uses a catheter to navigate through blood vessels (particularly tortuous abdominal aneurysms), it is being expanded to cannulate additional structures [2].

R. Rana (✉) · E. Liu
Michael G. DeGroote School of Medicine, McMaster University, Hamilton, ON, Canada
e-mail: ruqqiyah.rana@medportal.ca; eva.liu@medportal.ca

S. Athreya, M. Albahhar (eds.), *Demystifying Interventional Radiology*, https://doi.org/10.1007/978-3-031-12023-7_22

Embolization

In addition to imaging, there are other realms of interventional radiology that are seeing massive advances in technique and application to patient care. For example, embolization techniques have been applied to improving function and symptom profile in patients suffering from painful chronic musculoskeletal conditions such as tendinopathy, adhesive capsulitis, and degenerative joint disease [3–8]. While the basis of the procedures is simple—to decrease inflammatory angiogenesis and subsequent painful innervation through embolization techniques—the approaches used are quite complex and involve both pharmacological and calibrated microsphere agents [3–8].

Augmented Reality and Artificial Intelligence

In their article "Future Trends and Technologies in Interventional Radiology: What to Expect," Makary and Cerne [1] explore the possibilities of virtual and augmented reality in IR by providing examples of what can be enhanced in common procedures. An interesting application of this technology could include super-imposing the vital signs of a patient onto radiographic images obtained within a critical intervention, allowing the practitioner to gain access to all pertinent information through a single plane of vision. In addition, augmented reality can allow the simultaneous imaging of needle or device placement during ultrasound and can even make possible the visualization of 3D holograms of previously invisible structures underneath procedural drapes [1].

Virtual Reality and Education

Virtual reality has been explored in the field of interventional radiology with respect to education and hands-on practical skill acquisition in a low-stakes simulated environment [9]. Virtual reality lends itself particularly well to improve procedural skills in the areas related to vascular intervention and can be useful for identifying vessel anatomy and manipulating radiographic images. Examples include catheterization, angioplasty and stent placement, and angiography [9]. Traditionally, learners may struggle with their initial usage of the basic interventional radiology equipment, including needles, guidewires, and catheters, and having to dual-task with manual equipment and imaging can prove an overwhelming task at first. Virtual reality can circumvent this challenge by introducing technically complex procedures in an entirely visual format, allowing the interventional radiology trainee to become immersed within the technical procedure without the added manual equipment [9].

Virtual Reality in Practice

Virtual reality also has a place in clinical practice and may be utilized by experienced interventional radiologists in addition to trainees new to the field [10]. By and large, this technology has the advantage of creating a realistic anatomically accurate scenario which can mimic the actual patient profile, allowing it to be used for preplanning before complex procedures and mapping relevant anatomical structures and landmarks [10]. It can also be used to improve hand–eye coordination and to practice specific components within larger procedures.

References

1. Mina S. Makary MD, Jack Cerne MD. Future trends and technologies in interventional radiology: what to expect. Diagn Imaging. 2021. https://www.diagnosticimaging.com/view/future-trends-and-technologies-in-interventional-radiology-what-to-expect. Accessed 1 Jan 2022.
2. Mascini L. Operate using live, 3D image-guided navigation of the inner body. Innovation origins: your sneak peak of the future. 2019. https://innovationorigins.com/operate-using-live-3d-image-guided-navigation-of-the-inner-body/.
3. Midulla M, Pescatori L, Chevallier O, Nakai M, Ikoma A, Gehin S, Berthod PE, Ne R, Loffroy R, Dake M. Future of IR: emerging techniques, looking to the future… and learning from the past. J Belg Soc Radiol. 2019;103(1):12.
4. Okuno Y, Matsumura N, Oguro S. Transcatheter arterial embolization using imipenem/cilastatin sodium for tendinopathy and enthesopathy refractory to nonsurgical management. J Vasc Interv Radiol. 2013;24(6):787–92. https://doi.org/10.1016/j.jvir.2013.02.033.
5. Okuno Y, Oguro S, Iwamoto W, Miyamoto T, Ikegami H, Matsumura N. Short-term results of transcatheter arterial embolization for abnormal neovessels in patients with adhesive capsulitis: a pilot study. J Shoulder Elb Surg. 2014;23(9):e199–206. https://doi.org/10.1016/j.jse.2013.12.014.
6. Okuno Y, Korchi AM, Shinjo T, Kato S. Transcatheter arterial embolization as a treatment for medial knee pain in patients with mild to moderate osteoarthritis. Cardiovasc Interv Radiol. 2015;38(2):336–43. https://doi.org/10.1007/s00270-014-0944-8.
7. Okuno Y, Iwamoto W, Matsumura N, et al. Clinical outcomes of transcatheter arterial embolization for adhesive capsulitis resistant to conservative treatment. J Vasc Interv Radiol. 2017;28(2):161–7. https://doi.org/10.1016/j.jvir.2016.09.028.
8. Iwamoto W, Okuno Y, Matsumura N, Kaneko T, Ikegami H. Transcatheter arterial embolization of abnormal vessels as a treatment for lateral epicondylitis refractory to conservative treatment: a pilot study with a 2-year follow-up. J Shoulder Elb Surg. 2017;26(8):1335–41. https://doi.org/10.1016/j.jse.2017.03.026.
9. Duarte ML, Assis AM, Guimarães Junior JB, Carnevale FC. Virtual reality in interventional radiology education: a systematic review. Radiol Bras. 2021;19(54):254–60.
10. Garg T, Loya MF, Shrigiriwar A. Virtual reality and its applications in interventional radiology. Acad Radiol. 2020;27(10):1495.
11. Interventional Radiology. InsideRadiology. 2018. https://www.insideradiology.com.au/interventional-radiology/. Accessed 1 Jan 2022.

Index